HOW TO HAVE YOUR WAY WITH MEN

ANTHONY F BADALAMENTI PhD

Copyright © 1995 by Anthony F. Badalamenti

All rights reserved. No part of this book may be reproduced or transmitted in any form or by any means, electronic or mechanical, including photocopy, recording or any information storage or retrieval system, without prior permission in writing from the author.

Library of Congress Catalog Card Number   95-092558
ISBN   0-9648590-0-9

Published by: **Scientific Support**
  Westwood, New Jersey

THIS BOOK
IS DEDICATED TO
THE VERY BEST IN YOUR LIFE

Preface

Men see women as marvels of nature who know more about the ways of the human soul than they do. A man senses in a woman's presence a voice of nature not in him. It makes his emotions come to attention with wonder and admiration for so richly expressing a part of the universe he has a lesser share in. A woman is a glimpse into a richness that takes hold of men and draws them into what she is. Men easily fall under the spell of women's inner life and once taken with their feminine sense of things they yearn for more.

Men wish to have for themselves the wealth of intuitive feeling and natural wisdom that they see in women. They often think that if they could only understand the beautiful way of that intriguing other gender, then they would know how to take possession of it. It is very important to men to discover the right action for making a connection with women. The value men set on the happiness that women bring to their lives is in their longing to find this precious information. This is one of those male ways that can greatly increase a woman's opportunity with men.

This book is about a part of the male makeup that is as intuitive to men as feelings are, in general, to women. It is a deeper part of men known to them mostly by the exciting energy it offers. That energy reveals the psychology of the male's desire and of his efforts to connect with the female. It tells a story on the female advantage in the unseen effects women have on men.

Here are the inner thoughts and feelings that come to men as they try, in the way most natural to them, to connect with you as women. Here are the things men wish for, the things they want to find and the concerns they will love you for resolving. The wishes of the male heart differ in some ways from the female's but they are just as strong and compelling. Learn to see how they long for you and you will soon have more of what you want.

This book grew from two sources. More than twenty years of work in psychiatric research made the author sensitive to how quickly women take to the inner meaning of things. The intimate first hand sense of the issues is from more than fifteen years of work in the world of singles. One source is deeply emotional, the other very practical. They come together to report on how the psychology of male attraction shows you how to have your way with men.

The shortfalls in how women and men long for each other made me feel that there is a better way. There is more and better love waiting for women. The more a woman understands a man's inner world when his wishes turn to her, the more certain she is to have her way with him. You can quickly improve your position with men by learning more about how their hopes flow into their actions.

Getting the Most from Your Reading

A selection of poetry or prose introduces each chapter in this book. They are chosen to begin to move your thoughts and feelings in a favorable direction. Some are especially profound and may entice you to return to them for a longer taste of the authors' meanings. The style of the text itself is chosen from among those that are known to do the work for the reader. It is a style that goes to your intuitive emotional world, waking it up and moving it toward the insights that improve your life with men. As you move from chapter to chapter it will rework your thoughts and sentiments into a readiness to have the material serve you as needed.

The text is peppered with anecdotal material. I included this to bring the material closer to the familiar world where you want to fare better. It is all genuine. Some of the people cited are friends, others are acquaintances. In all cases I use names that are fictitious.

Each chapter concludes with an exercise or two. Please do them. They are based on the potent technique of visualization, a well evolved method that quickly brings about deep and long lasting change. The exercises will make the material come alive in your own experiences. They will make the ideas so live and breathe in you that you will bring them to all your next encounters without need of reflection or second sight.

I suggest that you read this book more than once. Find those areas that you most want to bring with you and reread the chapters that speak to them. Take the exercises with you and use them when you come upon situations that you want to work better for you. The exercises will put you in touch with how to create what you want. In time you will find yourself shaping the exercises to your life and success upon success will follow. Bon appetit!

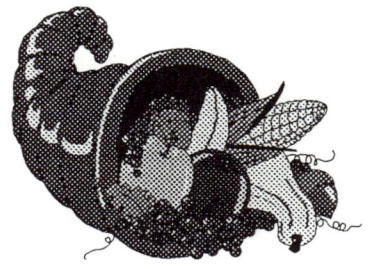

TABLE OF CONTENTS

Chapter 1. The Great Male Hope page 9
Chapter 2. Key To His World page 15
Chapter 3. Harmony and Melody page 23
Chapter 4. Things Men Love page 33
Chapter 5. Flirting & The Great Male Hope page 41
Chapter 6. The First Date page 47
Chapter 7. Working The Relation page 55
Chapter 8. Your Love and His Liberty page 63
Chapter 9. Ghosts from the Past page 71
Chapter 10. Ambivalence page 77
Chapter 11. Breaking Up page 85
Chapter 12. Aftermath and After page 93
Chapter 13. Avoidable Men page 101
Chapter 14. Things Men Dream About page 109
Chapter 15. The Women Men Fear page 119
Chapter 16. Sex page 127
Chapter 17. Lady Godiva page 135
Chapter 18. Knowing How Men See You page 141

Chapter 1.

The Great Male Hope

Remember the old saying,
"Faint heart ne'er won fair lady."

...from Don Quixote, part III, book 10
by Miguel de Cervantes

Every man far enough past puberty knows why he feels such excitement over having a woman in his life. She is a promise of joys and fulfillments he cannot reach by himself alone. Men sense from the earliest days of their attraction to women that those wonderful creatures improve the quality of life as nothing else can. For all of life men look with admiration at how beautiful is the promise that nature has put in every one of them. That is one reason why men, even very faithful men, never stop looking.

The attraction begins in those days of puberty when some unknown but welcome force creates in the boy something new, fresh and beguiling. The energies that once went to baseball and to teasing girls yield to a far greater good. Its object is unmistakable. The complacent know it all ways of only a month ago are overtaken by a new mystery in life — girls and how to get to them.

It is a marvel to watch, especially for adults who know its meaning better.

It is very tempting for boys to try to win girls' affections the same way they try to win at baseball, football and other sports. From the beginning males make a fundamental mistake in their strategies with the other sex. They assume that there is some objective action they can take to get to their goals. It does not take very long at all for this to lead to head scratching over why it does not work. What does that too-good-to-be-true Susie want me to do? This kind of question is a headline of sorts for boys in puberty.

From youth to old age, with and without feminism, a man knows that most women want him to take the initiative. It is a good idea to do so because his make up favors action. It is sometimes comical to watch how uninformed the actions most men take with women can be. The male continues to search for the "right" action to take. He almost never comes to question his assumption about there being such an action in the first place. He should question it. If he did he would learn that he could fare much better by looking at the nature of his actions rather than their intended outcomes.

The inner emotional and intuitive action that men need to take upon themselves is familiar to women but men rarely get to see it. A woman's key to certain success with men is to learn how to send that inner action to them. Men cling to their assumption of a correct action "out there" because it is their nature to do so. Men soon find that their inner conviction of what they assume to be true puts them in a quandary.

His insides tell him two things loudly and clearly. One is that life is never better than with one of them in your life. The other is that if you want one of them in your life get in gear and go for it. But how? A male's actions go out to the world with little supporting insight into what the female is looking for in the way of a right statement or message. There is a lack of correspondence between the measure taken by the male and the measure that the female wants.

Disappointment is common for both sexes during puberty. The male wonders what he failed to do correctly and assumes that she won't tell him. He will feel that way even if she does tell him where to find his treasured formula for success. He leaves the scene feeling that he cannot answer his own questions, try as he may. And so a feeling of helplessness before their desire for women arises in men. This is a very big issue in men's lives.

There is a rich sense of humor in the better side of human nature. Men use it to put wit and whimsy in their befuddlement. Men have favorite quips for making light of their concerns. A favorite is in the appeal to the law of large numbers. It means what it says: persist long enough with enough females and by chance success will follow. The comic spirit of having to wait a long time for something that should happen much sooner is in there. Men often gesture comically among themselves with arms out wide and a look up to heaven, exclaiming "What?" The meaning of "What?" is that men often feel powerless before their own wishes. When a woman's charms undo a man's composure, his first wish will be for the wisdom that tells how to put her into his life.

Our culture has created a colorful lore for making light of these things. It shows and tells with a smile. A hopeful but confused man sings in My Fair Lady "Why can't a woman be more like a man?" The value men place on women makes some of them take the spirit of Cervantes's words to heart by calling their wishes "the impossible dream". Men love to sustain themselves with humor when they find that their actions are not yet taking them to their hopes. This gives them fresh energy to make another go of it.

It pays to share their laughter and not just for the humor of it all. Men feel that the communication is good when you laugh with them. That will make them feel that they know what to do with their hopes for you.

The Great Male Hope
Exercise for Chapter 1.

Part I. This exercise will put you in touch with the earliest expressions of how men hope to discover the right action. Go back in your life to the time of puberty. Let some images flow into your consciousness. Look among them until you see a flirtation involving yourself or another girl, whichever you find more comfortable. Now draw the image in close so that you easily hear its sounds and see its movements. Draw it so close that the emotions involved come upon you. Now put yourself in the middle of the picture and focus on the boy in the scene. Go deeper still into the picture by stepping into his image. Take on his feelings as the flirtation moves from beginning to end.

What is he seeing and feeling as he enters the scene? What is taking place in him as it unfolds? How does he feel about its ending? Hold the images and let them flow through you. When you are finished repeat this for the girl. What are the major emotional differences for the boy and the girl? Stay with these feelings and images for a while. When you feel that they are releasing you, go on to Part II below.

Part II. Read again the quotation from Cervantes given above. Go with the image it stirs in you and note your feelings. Now see yourself again as the boy in Part I and repeat what you did there. How do the experiences of the boy and girl feel now as compared to your last visualization?

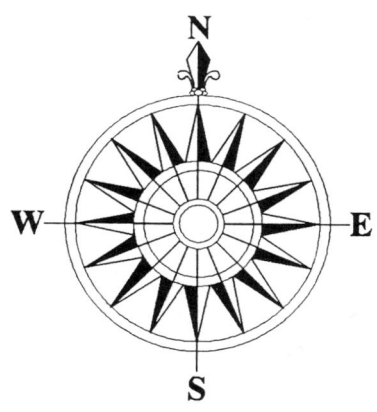

The Great Male Hope

Chapter 2.

Key To His World

*Suit the action to the word,
the word to the action;
with this special observance,
that you o'erstep not the modesty of nature.*

...from Hamlet by William Shakespeare

There is a beautiful and sensitive painting in the Metropolitan Museum of Art. It is The Storm by Cot, a nineteenth century work. The artist portrays a young couple running side by side through a wood just as a storm is about to break. They are moving to the viewer's left. The male has his right arm and the female her left arm extended up and outward holding a cloth over their heads which puffs out behind them as they dash along. His left arm is around her waist and her right arm up and over his left shoulder, both lovingly. He leads her by just a little as they seem to move together. Both are leaning forward as they move toward some sheltered haven your imagination tells you is there beyond the painting. The artist has created a wonderful image of loving cooperation. Cot's work tells a great deal about the way men see the women they choose to be with.

Men have their own version of the often expressed female wish to have a relation with a woman in a man's body. It's not the obvious word play — that would miss a man's sense of things. It is the wish to *enjoy shared activity* in their relations with women. What is shared is immaterial. It could be bicycle riding, a lecture, a trip, or something more emotional like a workshop or a movie. The event does not matter. **Doing it together is what counts.** Doing it together is what makes a man feel connected to you. Shared activity is a natural expression of what men feel and is also their way of exchanging meanings with others.

Most men do not feel that taking the lead in a relation speaks well for them or for the relation. Taking the lead is a great deal of emotional work for either person. Men see, as women do, that doing so cuts the flow of energy and good feelings between each other. They would rather share it. Men, in general, do not feed into the idea of being the male protector. Giving male strength and support, the directed and purposeful kind, through their presence is what they really want. It is an active way of sending their variety of love and care to the relation.

These things are rooted in the way a man sees life and the world. For him it is more a place in which to put deeds. Men are comfortable taking action by themselves or in concert with others. They feel natural and well with the world when actively doing things. For a woman the world is more a place in which to put feelings that create or draw events to themselves. Women put their meanings into feelings and emotions. They also use emotions to signify acts and to tell their meanings. Men do it the opposite way — they use acts to *signify feelings*. This is why doing together is important to men. Doing together tells them what is happening. A man wants shared activity because that is his major way of knowing what is going on in the relation. In fact, it is his major way of knowing what is going on, period.

Men do not discover meaning with intuitive feelings as easily as women. They try to read the deed, so to speak. They unconsciously assume that women also show meaning more in deeds than in feelings. For women it runs the other way. They count feelings in more than deeds for telling them where meaning lies and they unconsciously assume that men do the same. A man mature enough to be in touch with his own inner life and who cares about a woman will also try to exchange meanings with her that way. Likewise, a mature woman, who cares and is in touch with her dynamic side, will try to read his meanings and to show her own in her actions.

Look at what he is doing when you wonder what is going on in a man or want to become clearer on his meanings. His emotions will tell some of the story but the entire message will be in the deeds he is putting before you. This is the opposite of what most women find natural — to have action follow feeling. It is worth musing over the way men value expressed actions. Men see a meaning in an action even though they savor the feelings that create it. Their feelings are more of a relish in the process of taking action than the main event itself. Understanding this will help you to become more successful with men.

Suppose that a shy man discovers you while in the middle of talking to his friends. He will tell you about his shy interest more by the way he acts out an intense involvement with his friends than any show of feeling. His make believe devotion to his dialogue with his friends will express his shy interest in you more than with any emotion you will sense coming from him. If he decides to try his luck with you he will soon withdraw his interest from his friends and seek you out. He will announce his interest by directing himself to you and to no one else. Key into his action if you want to learn more about him. Give him emphasis on speaking over sending feeling and you will make him feel that you favor his purpose. He will take your words and movements toward him to tell of your interest and he will sense less of it in your emotions.

A man will feel that you are connecting with him when you show an empathy for his actions and what they mean to him. This is one area where he will read your feelings. Doing so will make him feel exempt from having to struggle to find how to put himself into what he says to win your interest. This is a large issue for most men. He will also feel grateful to you for connecting with him and will want to give you more of himself because you know his meanings.

I had a recent experience rich in imagery of how men see meaning in action. I was having lunch with my friend John. We were seated near a three foot high brick divider separating us from a lovely garden walkway in the ground floor of an office building. All of a sudden a woman, whose name I later recalled was Linda, presented herself to us with a welcome smile across the divider. I half recognized her and said to her "Don't I know you?" and before I could say anymore she was engaging John whom it turns out she used to work with. I found her attractive and wondered how I struck her.

Linda made several obvious asides to me in talking to John and I noted her interest. It was easy to see that Linda had that active streak in her personality that makes it so easy for men to know her message. She made it a point to ask John if he frequently came there for lunch and I could feel her side energy coming to me. Linda finished by bidding us good day and sending a directed expression to me as she left. I came away thinking how nice it would be to get to know her better.

I knew that she would be easy and fun to get to know because of the way she puts herself and her meanings into to her expressed actions.

Key To His World
Exercise for Chapter 2.

Part I. Recall some times in your life when you watched, or took part in, boys and men doing things together. Some sporting events or images of men working together to make something may come to mind. Look carefully and come to what is natural and easy in the way they do what they do. How much do they communicate with words as opposed to gestures that they just seem to know the meaning of? Stay with it until you see that they are held together by the common purpose of wanting to get something accomplished.

Part II. This part will help to see what your feelings are on shared activity. Spend a few minutes becoming quiet within. Muse over scenes of play with boys and girls from before puberty. Pick one that you like. Use visualization to make the scene come alive in the present: draw the images closer to yourself, deepen the colors, amplify the sounds, brush against the surfaces and so on. Feel the life of the scene near you and around you.

Move into the picture and see it as a participant. Look at the boy or boys you are playing with. Step into yourself and take on your feelings from that time. What is it like for you? Pause now to let your feelings and images work their way into you. Stay there until you feel that you want to move on.

Return to the boy(s) you were playing with. Step into him and his feelings. Feel his glee over playing with you and the others. What does it mean to him? If this is difficult to feel then look for an action he hopes will connect with you and the others. Repeat this exercise with material from later in your life. What is different for you and the male at the different times?

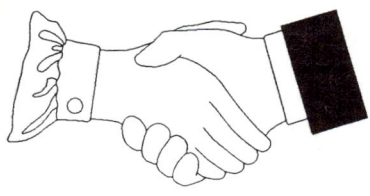

Key To His World

Chapter 3.

Harmony and Melody

The fountains mingle with the river
And the rivers with the Ocean,
The winds of Heaven mix for ever
With a sweet emotion;
Nothing in the world is single;
All things by a law divine
In one spirit meet and mingle.
Why not I with thine?—

...from Love's Philosophy by Percy Bysshe Shelley

Sexual differences are like green and red maple trees in most ways. There is no major difference between the maples except for their leaf colors. Male versus female is similar. Each sex has most of the natural goods of the other, with the proportions reversed and a splash of their gender's color thrown in. A woman has more of richly intuitive and emotional capacities than a man. A man has a quicker sense than women for making logical plans and for putting action out into the world. Where she is better with emotional commitment, he is better with committed purpose.

A major difference is with intuition versus action. Men also intuit emotional meanings and express their feelings but not so richly as women and women send their actions into the world but not so vigorously or readily as men. Men show overdone sympathy for emotional spells in women because they have less feeling and intuitive ability. They put into women their own difficulties in dealing with feeling issues and assume that women are as undone by their emotions as men are. Women may welcome this kind of attention but they easily see it as naive and often overdone.

Most men feel that women show too much sympathy for their, the men's, shortfalls and failures in life. Women feel that men's disappointments in action are as disturbing to them as to themselves because their makeup is first to an intuitive sense and second to action. Men usually feel more able, and willing, than women think to shake off the setbacks in their actions, however disappointing they may be, and to quickly regroup and try again.

Nature has spelled out clearly that the kinds of initiative fall of themselves upon now one and then upon the other member of the couple. Nature wants the leadership role to be mobile in the relation, a wish that men generally favor more than women. What faces the couple should be free to command one or the other, as fitting, for the leadership in the relation. This is something that men prize greatly in a relation and women can make the couple prosper by giving themselves to it.

When the couple needs to get a sense of other people's inner lives then it falls more naturally to the female. When it is to make objective plans for action and to then carry them out, then it falls more to the male. Each partner's lesser capacity goes out to harmonize with the lead given by the other's greater ability. Put differently, the leadership role changes the couple's melody and the greater part of that change is led by the sex better fit to first go to what is before them. The richer partner has the good feeling of making the other's way easier and of supporting that other's growth. As this position moves from one to the other, so do the joys of giving and getting.

When things go smoothly a woman's feelings put a joy and exuberance into a man that make him feel life is simply wonderful. Men put a sense of centeredness and trust into a woman making her feel that he has found her and that the relation is here for her. Both feel that life is sending them good things but not entirely in the same way. Men are very much aware of the blessings women bring them but they don't often sense what they do for women. It seems that women, with the advantage of knowing from within, have a commanding lead over men in understanding the relation. They feed patient emotion to the male's comprehension of the tie that joins them together and she welcomes his openness to her support. The way he focuses her inner experience is satisfying for the woman.

The positive differences that create and bind the relation also set the stage for challenges to it. Men bring with their yen for shared action a naivete for the feeling part of it. Women bring with their love of fulfillment and mutual growth an often naive sense of what the action principle in men is about emotionally. Meaning offered in action can puzzle a woman and action delivered in feeling can utterly baffle a man. The meaning rich cues for leadership that go out so easily from each partner are not always so easily received by each other.

Men often wish for a more tangible grounding to some of the woman's perceptions. Men *want* to discover more of the emotional meaning of their experience than women usually assume. Insight helps to orient men in the logical ways they find natural and comfortable. It provides welcome relief from the feeling of emotional uncertainty they often have with women. This is an unpleasant feeling that they experience as distancing. Men also want to uphold woman's actions and purpose more than women assume. That wish is comfortable with men's readiness to take action. Men want women to accept the natural shifts in who leads the couple because they will make the couple work better.

Men love to see in their first encounter with a woman her yen to do for herself. They see this as a making a statement on involvement via shared action on her part. They also see it as predicting a communication they will relish. Men take that yen as telling of great goodness to be found in a relation with her. It gives men a rush of feeling that two is better, far better, than one. Men want to work together in relations with women more than most women realize. A man feels that he *knows* what is happening between himself and the woman he cares for when they are working together.

The flow of good feelings and energy in the relation can be stunted when women offer too much of their intuitive emotional strengths. This can make a man feel as though he is standing on the outside and blocked in his purpose. He is also likely to be confused and to feel unable to keep up with the richer part of her nature. He may not consciously know what it all means but he will sense that he cannot keep up and doesn't know why he is being asked to. This situation offers him little place for the logical and active ways that come so easily to men.

Modest doses of your emotional richness will make the communication between you prosper. This is especially true early on. Men need measured amounts of the deep and easy sensitivity of women to the psychology of it all. Men do better with samples than with the entire menu. It takes a little preparation for the sexual differences in feeling versus acting to meet and form around the common good of the relation.

Figuring out what women want is an issue of much concern for most men. Men wonder, usually more unaware of their thoughts than aware, how to work the communication from one sex to the other. They do not understand women's wishes as clearly as they can or should and often miss the meaning of her expressions. The more a wish becomes an expressed act the more a man will see its meaning. He will then feel positive about making an effort to realize it for her. Men feel secure when they know what is asked of them and can prepare to deliver it. Women feel secure when they sense that the men in their lives will uphold them. Putting it another way, each gender wants and needs more of the other has. The male needs more wisdom and the female needs to be more demonstrative.

I watched a couple thrive as they accepted the natural shifts in its leadership role. When they first met Jean was taken with Ron's dynamic and often bold ways and he was drawn to her soft and misty side. As she became more comfortable with Ron's kind of energy in herself she became more peppy and engaging. He liked this and found that he wanted to slowly give more of the lead for emotional energy over to her. At the same time he discovered in himself some of Jean's gentler and more intuitive ways. She was delighted to give him more and more liberty to take the lead with feeling issues and quiet understanding. The growth behind these shifts created more of the way of the other in each of them and made them closer.

It went the other way with another couple, Alan and Cathy. She favored his boyish honesty and upbeat ways. Alan liked Cathy's daring do, especially in the outdoors. She often took the lead and saw how he followed with relish. In time he took in her daring ways and wanted to express them in the lead. She sensed this and the playful lead slowly moved more from Cathy to Alan. His upbeat ways infected her with a brighter and more perky outlook. The energy for optimism and hopefulness then took root in her. They did well together.

Harmony and Melody
Exercise for Chapter 3.

Part I. Here is an exercise to help you with the experience of giving and getting the leadership role with a male. Recall a piece of music that you like and play it through your mind long enough to spot where there is harmony and melody. Harmony occurs where one or more voices or instruments add their sound to the music without changing it. Melody occurs when a voice or instrument enters and alters some or all of the composition. Stay with it until you can hear the difference. It's alright if you get lost in the music for a while, as long as you get to sense the difference.

Part II. Now recall some recent times when you were with a fellow, whether for meeting, dating or commitment. Settle on a scene that has emotional meaning for you, one that is rich with color and intensity. Let it move easily and freely across your conscious mind. As it does so note who has the harmony and who has the melody — who follows and who introduces fresh material. You may also want to note if the roles are natural and appropriate for you and your partner.

Whatever role you had in the original scene use the visualization methods to enter the role of the other.

This will sensitize you to his experience in both leading and following. If your position was leading in your memory then find another one in which you also follow and repeat the exercise.

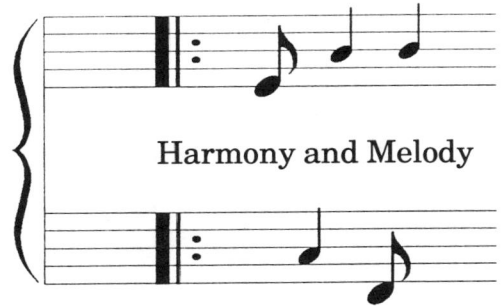

Chapter 4.

Things Men Love

*O what could be nice
Than her ways with a man?*

...from Light Listened by Theodore Roethke

Is anything more obvious than a man's eye falling upon a woman? It is hard for men to stifle that very basic level of attraction but second sight comes quickly to most of them. Their eyes move gingerly with their thoughts looking for other, more subtle qualities in a woman's personality and ways. Not finding them, the attraction soon fades leaving little behind but the hopes that the first attraction brought to mind. The things that attract men to women are far deeper and more emotionally charged than most women realize.

A man's second view of a woman comes very soon after the first, certainly in less than several minutes. The second one is the one that counts because he will commit his energies on its basis. In a make believe world where all wishes are met and fulfilled a woman would have the right physical parameters together with the right subtleties of mind and spirit. For most men an intriguing fact follows after and replaces this ideal fiction. Few women seem to be aware of it and even fewer work it to their advantage. The fact is that a woman's winning ways — those emotional goods that work wonders on a man's sense of feeling good to be alive — radically alter a man's perception of how she looks. Accommodations set in as a man comes to care. At the moment of first meeting a man is estimating just how much her sweet and subtle ways can take hold of him and make everything else about her seem right. I do not personally know any men who have told this to the women they have known, but I feel that this useful fact is worth noting.

The male's lesser ability to deal with his feelings is behind these things. Here, in their weaker area, they want to be overtaken by a woman's ways, to have her beguile him into a richer and fuller emotional life. Men want women to put their feelings into them, making them feel vibrant and more alive. A woman who is in touch with these things can be very far from a man's physical ideal and still connect very well with him. From the first meeting and through every phase of the relation, a man will value your power to put captivating energy before him to enchant him into drawing nearer to your inner beauty and power.

There are hints that nature redeemed men's feeling function somewhere along the line. Men have an exquisitely sensitive ability to see how well a woman can put the desired emotional difference in them. Her emotional abilities, in his eyes, can free him from many inhibitions to giving himself to her. The persistent inner voice telling of physical requirements for his female partner is a nuisance most men would like to be relieved of. A woman who can stir a man's inner life of emotions, feelings and sensations can easily put him past this pest and take her pick from the many.

Men value seductiveness but they prize cooperation more highly. A woman who lends her spirit has the most winning way in men's eyes. Men want more from a woman than to enjoy her loving ways and to be near to those wonderful differences. A woman who will be partner to playing the game of life promises a man an excitement and a richness of meaning he cannot find elsewhere. Men sense that the greatest joy and energy are to be found in the company of a playful spirit, even though sexy ways never fail to get their first attention. Men want women who will play in earnest and join them in becoming two moving around one another. You could say with much accuracy that the search for a sexy pal is a great wish in men.

Cooperation makes life easier and clearer, a state men prefer and a playful, spunky spirit is a turn on, even to women. Add to these sexy and genuine and you have a highly fetching formula for drawing men in. Sexy speaks for itself. Genuineness is in many ways a richer and more distinctive quality. It sends out a charming and beguiling message telling a man that she is easy to be with because there are no hidden messages he needs to decode. Genuine means that she is what she appears and that the prospect of wanting to meet and perhaps study the possibilities is real. It makes a man breathe easy and feel that he need only follow her open, authentic leads to win her favor.

Genuineness also inspires a sense of respect for her person because it speaks for self esteem, that robust sense of self that puts a come-be-with-me charm in her expressions and actions. The more a woman manifests healthy self esteem, the more men assume that she is easy to be with. Men sense at once that such a woman is better prepared to reveal freely, but with dignity, who and what she is. In other words, the better a woman feels about herself, the easier it is for her to make it easier for the man wishing to try his luck with her.

This brings to mind a good friend. She is a young woman who has all four of the above — she is cooperative, playful, sexy and genuine. Her personality style has that active flair which makes it easy for men to communicate with her. She meets them half way by sending action messages along with feeling messages. The limitations to her appearance would make you think that she has less success with men than she truly does. The fact is, she is highly successful. Her winning ways send energy into men that charm them into moving eagerly her way. Her winning personal ways are a melt down to the inner limitations men feel and she frees them from having to do any inner work in the process. You could easily say that men feel it is a stroke of good luck to meet her and see her way for themselves. They certainly like what she does to them and for them. She makes them feel warm, alive, uplifted and natural to be with her.

She puts the shoe on the other foot by making women, often far more eye catching than herself, wonder what she is doing right. Her energy tells men easily and clearly what she wants from them by eliciting it from them. She wants from men what all women want — to be discovered. She sends with her message of what she wants the acknowledgment of knowing what men want, and in the style they understand. Men perceive her to be the accessible woman she is. In giving such large free samples of her good inner things so generously and easily she creates a rush of excited good feelings in men that magnetizes them to her.

Things Men Love
Exercise for Chapter 4.

Call to mind flirtations you have seen but have not been a part of. Select one where an attractive women does not achieve her goal. If you know of none in real life then turn to movies you have seen. Draw the image in close so that you can see her facial movements as she speaks and his expressions in response to what she says. Follow the image from the beginning of the encounter to its natural end. What does she do and say that piques his initial interest? How does he express his interest and lead her into further self disclosure? At what point and why does he begin to lose interest? If you wanted this to go well what would you do differently?

Now call to mind a second flirtation that went well and repeat the above. At what point and how does she secure his ongoing interest? Go into her feeling state at that critical moment where his interest in her is anchored and hold it for a while. What differences in the second woman account for her success? What was more comfortable about the second experience?

Things Men Love

Chapter 5.

Flirting & The Great Male Hope

Somewhere she waits to make you win,
Your soul in her firm white hands;
Somewhere the gods have made for you
The woman who understands.

...from The Woman Who Understands
by Everard Jack Appleton

Men bring the feeling of hope to their encounters with women. They come to the moment wishing for, but not really expecting, their offer of cooperative action. If you could look within men at such times you would find romantic images of knights and warriors who are ready to endure great trials for the hand of their fair lady. Men take pause to reflect, breathe deeply and gird up their loins before they sally forward to try their luck.

They take action on their hopes feeling like pilots flying at night in the early days before radar. They are anxious that they will not know, and may never learn, what right thing to do to win the favor they seek. The woman who understands and accepts this is in a position of informed advantage. She can help him win her interest by helping him to give her what she wants. These are moments where a woman's romantic interest and inner wisdom can work together to realize her hopes and his.

This is an area that wants measured care from both the man and the woman. Neither sex has entirely the same priorities as the other. The interaction is rife with many levels of false equating of one's wishes with the other's needs. Apples are offered where oranges are wanted. The efforts here are suggestive of an American and a Russian trying to find an area of agreement by speaking to each other only in their native tongues. It is probably the element of humor in the large gap between the offered actions and their intended meaning that saves the moment and keeps enough effort alive to eventually get to the goal. The situation is an opportunity for whichever sex, or both, chooses to go after it with eyes for what is really going on.

The poetry quoted captures the nature of the woman's opportunity. The understanding his nature is asking for is that his meaning and intentions are sent to you in what he says and does. He comes to you with the wish to send his energy to you. Because he is a male his feelings will not carry his meaning as richly as yours would as a woman. The heart of the opportunity is in seeing that you already have his intention to give you what you want. It is for you to decode his actions into what they mean on your feeling, intuitive level. You can then begin to tell him in active ways what else you want. Adopt his idiom and be direct, while being warm and interested.

Look at the meaning of your emotions in the moments of exchange. Watch to see if you are unconsciously relying on him to grasp your meaning through your feelings the way you would if you were with another woman. He won't get much of the message that way unless he is unusual or atypical. Move from sending your meaning emotionally to sending it in words, gestures and acts. What kind of acts? Whatever fits his disposition.

Suppose the person you have just met at a party is a man who likes to keep his own counsel, a thing that you can see in how he expresses himself. Show that you know his meaning by suggesting that you both move to a more private spot. He will consciously take that to mean that you are reasonable — men love that — and not simply that you are considerate and courteous. Its unconscious meaning to him will be that he can communicate with you. He will see it that way because you have followed the meaning of his expressed actions.

As second example, suppose you have met someone who soon has you dancing with him but you sense that his heart is not in it. Whatever the real meaning of dancing is for him, you don't yet know it. Ask him to fetch you something to nibble or drink so that you can leave the dance floor to pause and chat. He will appreciate the offered relief and feel you are reasonable and considerate.

Unconsciously he will feel that you have properly read that the meaning of his act (dancing) was to tell you how much he wanted to learn what you are like to be with and to seize the opportunity of you before the others could.

When you work with him for the success of his expressed action, you are also securing your own wishes. If you pursue a relation later, you can work on making more effort come your way by having him get more in touch with your expressed emotional meanings. Once he feels that you can read his meanings he will be eager to learn how to read yours. As his affection for you grows, so will the importance of your meanings.

Flirting & The Great Male Hope
Exercise for Chapter 5.

Part I. This will help to sensitize you more to what men bring to their first meetings with you. Recall an episode where a fellow showed obvious first interest in you but then did not sense your interest. Use the visualization technique to replay the event from start to finish.

Go to its beginning and step into his experience. Become him. Stay with it and come to feel his emotional response to what unfolds. Now recall several more such episodes and repeat this for each one. What are you experiencing as you try one, then another? Hold this experience as you go to part II.

Part II. Still as the male in the last visualization, see him approaching you. What is the meaning of what he says and does as he tries to win your interest? Go with his actions more than with your own emotions and connect with him by showing him that you see the meanings of what he does. Give him some confirming action such as a hand touch, a telling facial gesture, a suggestion to share a snack, a yen to see something interesting where you are, and so on.

Do this until your visualization tells you that he is confident of winning enough interest from you to show you more of himself. What is his inner experience like when he sees confirming interest coming from you in an expressed action?

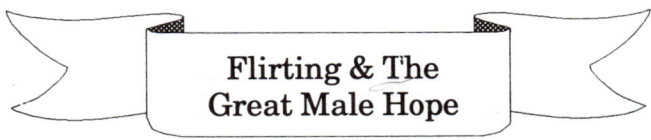
Flirting & The Great Male Hope

Chapter 6.

The First Date

Like everybody who is not in love, he imagined that one chose the person whom one loved after endless deliberation and on the strength of various qualities and advantages.

...from Remembrance of Things Past. Cities of the Plain, pt. I by Marcel Proust

He calls as promised and you arrange a first date. Many men do not place the promised call and you wonder why. The conscious reason is usually an honest reassessment of what he saw when with you, turning his sense of where greater good lies into not pursing it further. At a deeper, unconscious level there is a need to see that energy and action are being well placed. If he feels at this level that your interest in him may lag then he will falter. He has an unconscious need to keep his energies flowing in order to get to his intended goals. *Unconscious doubt* will seek to rescue his flow of energy from a depressive blocking by giving him the conscious pause that results in his not calling you. Put differently, it's not you, it's him.

A man brings some anxiety to his first date with a woman about keeping alive her interest in him. His desirability is on the line and, if you have really struck his fancy, he will be eager to not commit any major blunders. In all circumstances he will bring to you his longstanding and distracting uncertainties about how to find what you want and to deliver it. His energy and attention will flow to getting a handle on your ways and how to appeal to them. This is a large area of concern with men, especially when they feel certain that you can put happiness in their lives. What energy is left over goes to learning more about you. Among all other things, this is an occasion for a woman to learn how he puts his uncertainties into expressed actions.

Suppose he tells you about a movie he recently saw and enjoyed. It had beautiful footage, fine acting and good direction. Yet for all the positives he still cannot see how the story line comes together. On a first date this decodes into his saying that he has anxious doubts about pleasing you. You can use this material to great advantage. Tell him that given *his* description of the flick you would feel the same way. He will take this to mean that you are telling him he can be certain about your good feelings for him. Story telling, of sorts, can be very handy for getting messages across.

The opening quote from Marcel Proust suggests that a man will come equipped with his awareness of a mental fiction that he thinks can light up his life. You can ignore it and put your energy into showing him your good inner stuff and the magical power of your feminine ways. You will know you are connecting if he starts to tell tales about going happily into the future. For example, he may begin to tell you about his intentions to travel to wonderful places where he is sure he will find revelations, marvels and "turn-ons". His intent to get you to volunteer that you will join him is transparent. Or he may ask for your view on how he could best spend his now available time, given several options that are clearly meant to include you. The message is on the tip of his nose. If you want him then go for it.

After you have given him your offer you should go directly to your natural emotional ways and send those good feelings his way. He will be primed to receive them. Why won't he ask outright, you wonder? The male action principle, seeking meaning in an act, will keep him from easily reading your eager *feelings* by themselves. If he did then he would ask outright. He needs to see your message put in an active form such as "You know, my time runs about the same as yours. Why not get together and..." Put your good inner stuff out to him in its familiar form and deliver it also with expressed words and actions. Do this if you feel you want to go further with him. You will see your success in the welcome drop of his anxious uncertainty about winning your good feelings.

Men will get your emotional messages, first date and elsewhere, if you put them also into some form of expressed action. The wisdom of doing it on the first date is in building his confidence that he can communicate with you. He wants to see in *his* way that you are picking up on him. Setting a frame like this with him will make him feel so warm and good about you that he will gladly work to learn more about what you want and how to give it to you. The richness of your opportunity is spun out well in the affirmation "The more you give, the more you get."

If you are reaching him then after his first date with you he will be spending time dealing with his apprehensions about getting involved. This is a strongly positive statement about you and not at all a negative. The more he finds you desirable the more he will have to confront his male ambivalence about giving up his search and settling down to develop a relation with one woman. You will have many forays with his ambivalence and you should learn to read them well. It is a good sign even though it is a source of anxiety and a nuisance to you.

If you suspect that a man is ambivalent it pays to give him a call. It will be an action message in his natural idiom that will get to him, one way or the other. A man's emotions will spontaneously salute you when you as a woman give him a message in his own terms.

If he wants you and needs a push to go for a relation then your call will very likely push him over the threshold.

The First Date
Exercise for Chapter 6.

Go back in your mind's eye to images from your very first date. Move closer to it and draw it in. Note the movements of gestures of the fellow you are with. Get closer so that you can see his mouth move as he speaks and the expressions in his legs and torso. What do you see in his groping about to link with you? What is his inner model for what a girl should be? Is he unduly anxious, perhaps stumped over how to send himself to you? Does he *realize* that your emotions are entering him? Run the scene from start to finish. Hold the image and step out of it.

Look at it now with communication in mind. He probably sent his messages with words and motions and you sent yours more with feelings and hints. Get in touch with the nature of the exchanges, good and otherwise. Rewind the scene to its beginning and return now to the images. Go close and step into yourself.

Replay the event with you sending messages in his natural style. Watch how his responses to you change and move closer to what you want.

The First Date

Chapter 7.

Working The Relation

I understand thy kisses and thou mine,
And that's a feeling disputation:
But I will never be a truant, love,
Till I have learn'd thy language;

...from King Henry IV—Part I
by William Shakespeare

The idea of work in a relation waits in the background of its honeymoon phase. Man and woman at this time are overjoyed to have found one another. It is a delightful period of bubbly energy, euphoric feelings and feeding off one another. There is little pause in eagerly getting to know one another. The couple's tempo slows as they discover that they are really there for one another. Women are first to pause in seeing this and men often pause sooner with anxiety over it.

A large part of a relation for the woman is interacting with his ambivalence over it. Women usually enter relationships prepared for this and remain alert for it to surface. A man usually comes to it hoping that she will resolve his ambivalence for him by sending her good inner self to him. A man wants to discover that the woman he is with is right for him. He even wants to think he discovered it by himself. Men's inner experience of ambivalence is not pleasant for them and most would like it to go away. It is wise for a woman to invest her goodness in this part of the fellow she cares about. He will be grateful to you for doing so and he will admire how your psyche does for him what he cannot do himself. *I usually feel their ambivalence. Instead I need to make it go away.*

Having one special person in their lives seems to come more easily to women than men, a fact that sits well with patiently melting away a man's mixed feelings. The root of men's ambivalence is not what most women think and fear. It is not that he is ever looking for a better option. That may be at times what he is *consciously* thinking but it is a red herring. The real, unconscious, meaning is that it makes him anxious to deal more closely with his feelings. His intuition that he is less able to *process* strong emotions than she is makes him anxious. He may then feel without control.

Perceptive women will give men positive energy to uplift them. They will move more slowly when sending out their wish for men to sense the meanings of their inner world. Men want to go at a slow and comfortable pace with her emotional power, especially early on in a relation.

As a man draws closer to you emotionally he will be looking more and more for the way of shared action because that is his natural and ready way to be, do and grow together. This contains the key to what intimate relations mean to a man. The highest expression of that shared action is in the wonder and joy of coming together sexually. It is an event that tells a man a great deal about a woman's readiness to act in concert.

This may sound like it has comic value but I mean it earnestly. Men want women who tell them what to do, literally. This means telling them in words and not sending subtle messages in the hope of his catching and decoding them. A man is innately ready to generalize from how well you share actions in lovemaking to how willing you are to do so elsewhere. It goes further than this. A man will unwittingly see your intimate cooperation in almost every other thing you do together. It is remarkable how his unconscious will go about putting that sweet and positive energy into the images of everything else you do.

These are things that will motivate a man to draw closer to you and to think less and less of other parts of life. As for that nuisance, the prospect of someone else, it pays for a woman to be firm. Taking a stand will make you more desirable in his eyes. Men respect the firmness of purpose that spells out the terms of a relation and they respond well to it. Just don't do it too early. The fact is, they want you to be firm because it makes them stand to and spares them the inner work of resolving their ambivalence.

Wait until you have enough signs that he wants to be there for you to let him know how important it is to you to get closer. A reasonable amount of time might easily be two or three months. Otherwise you will make him unduly anxious when you want him to feel good about what is important to you and to respect your purpose.

Hinting at less outflow of your goodness to him can go a long way with a hesitant man who really does care about you. He will quickly make the logical leap going from your hint at how good he has it now to the prospect of not having it so good in the future. If he is sensitive he will even begin to have images of losing you whirl around his head. I do not recommend putting out a threat unless your own frustration tells you that it wise to do so.

A man's fear of closeness goes away slowly. The more he can read your meanings in your expressed actions the happier he will be. He well feel that you understand him and make things easy for him. He will conclude, emotionally and mentally, that he wants to be with you more and get closer to you. If your nearness to him, or its suggestion, makes him anxious deal with it through an action. How do you do that? Tell him, in words, that you see that getting closer makes him uncomfortable and ask him how he wants to manage it. He will respect your for asking him to do something about it. He will also be grateful for "giving him permission" to deal with his difficult feelings out in the open.

Men have conversations with each other all the time about such things. They help because talking puts the anxious feeling into an act and men know how to deal with acts. When men do this they do not send each other deep feelings and neither should you. They just support each other's anxiety over dealing with feeling issues. Giving intuitive (silent) emotional support to a man in this situation will make him more anxious. Give him something that supports action such as joking with him. You could suggest, and with a grin, that the relation might be fatal for him or that you will drop him from your will if he lets you down or whatever wit you favor.

Men will love you for making light of their anxieties in relations. They are forever struggling with society's expectation of them to be creatures that make things happen in life. When you tease them about such matters they feel that you are one with them in spirit and they will want more of you in their lives.

Men can misread your making light of things as just being silly. A woman's silliness is a free and joyful of expression of some of her best inner life. Men really do want women to be silly but it has to come off right. When she is silly she tells him of a natural goodness he should take note of because it belongs to the better part of life. It is pure *joie de vivre* telling him of what is and can be when he draws near to you.

A man may look at it from an action point of view. He could unconsciously see it as opposing the strong, focused purpose needed to get things done. He cannot help seeing it as going in a direction unfavorable to his makeup and his purpose. Little do men realize that most women will only be silly when they care and trust enough to do so. They are quick to give that carefree energy to one another but they think long and hard before giving it to a man.

Give him your silliness and let him know its meanings. Tell him with and without words that this goes only to those you care for in a special way. Tell him that in your play the real and important part of you, the part that gives love and laughter and meaning to life, is *going to him*. The act of telling him will bring your meaning to him and afterwards he will enjoy your glee so much more.

Working The Relation
Exercise for Chapter 7.

Pick a moment of deep interest from a relation. It could be a current one or one from the past. Recreate it using the familiar methods of visualization. Look into it and come to why you find it interesting. Hold your thoughts and images close to yourself. Now enter the scene and step into the male. Let the scene roll forward in time and take his experience and perception of it. What is different? What is his experience telling you about the important part of it? Do you sense parts of his experience that he would rather keep to himself?

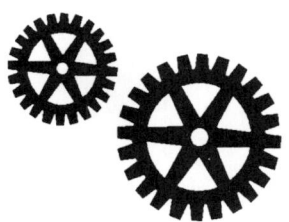

Working The Relation

Chapter 8.

Your Love and His Liberty

How do I love thee? Let me count the ways.
I love thee to the depth and breadth and height
My soul can reach, when feeling out of sight
For the ends of Being and ideal Grace.

...from Sonnets from the Portuguese, no. 43
by Elizabeth Barrett Browning

I must down to the seas again,
to the lonely seas and the sky,
And all I ask is a tall ship
and a star to steer her by,
And the wheel's kick and the wind's
song and the white sail's shaking,
And a gray mist on the sea's face
and gray dawn breaking.

...from Sea Fever by John Masefield

This chapter is about a part of life so emotionally charged that it wants a voice from both sides. I put two quotes in its beginning, one to announce each side's position, with the idea of balance in mind.

Some say that women's monogamous hearts and men's polygamous drives are behind it all. This is a droll idea often met with ripples of laughter and cynical smiles. It amuses but does not tell of the nature of things. In the mind of nature the distinct energies of the couple are there to fuel a path to a wiser and happier life for both.

Is there a woman who does not see her higher purpose as sending the wonder of her inner life out to do marvels in the world? If for all of time poets, playwrights and artists salute this magical inner world and the way it creates the outer world then who can see it otherwise? Women are creatures of the deep and they are subtle and sweeping in their ways. The object of their ways is to create and sustain life itself, not only new life, but all life. It is fundamental in women to want to have that long, sustained and patient relation with her love that forever after goes on giving it more life.

The image of telepathy is fitting for how a woman acts on what she loves. Her energy and her ways are barely visible but their effects are known by the wonders they produce. Men know this below conscious awareness where the same part of nature also lives in them. In her relation with the man she cares for, she wants to create and uphold what he is and can become. She wants her expressions to give him more of the life of the universe that she has more of to begin with. These good things have driven poets and artists in every age to reach to the limits of words and forms to capture what she sends to others.

It is in the nature of what a woman gives for her to seek a close, consistent and ongoing relation. These things are true for everything a woman comes to love. A woman needs a man in her life to live out these fulfillments. The kind of presence she wants and needs is well expressed in the quoted words of Elizabeth Barrett Browning. There is a lofty and eternal quality to a woman's love, different in some ways from a man's.

There is in every man a restless energy that wants to go out into the world, not in the deeply personal and misty way of women, but in a dynamic way that reshapes it. Men are driven to rework the world, literally. The objects of a man's energy come and go. They could be home repair, designing a computer, taking risks in a business venture, and so on. It is not in the nature of the objects of masculine energy to engage men for very long periods of time, a point where the way of male and female energy parts. Men need to be ready to send their effort to fresh objects as they offer themselves. Such events can occur almost anytime.

Male energy is ready to vigorously remove what stands in the way of its object. This is very easy to see in the dark side of some nasty figures in human history. In health and higher purpose, it is easy to see in road and building construction, creating new business activity, and ocean and space exploration and so on.

The male principle in nature attracts things that must be met boldly, often with adventure and always with enterprise. I like that!

Both energies live in both sexes but not in the same proportions. The fitness of different energies for the couple's needs announces itself gently and obviously. Working with the tune of the different energies is a shared activity bringing joy and fulfillment to the couple. A woman's major theme follows lines of long term devotion and patient commitment. The man's are more mobile and restless, poised to swiftly assume fresh directions.

A man feels within himself a hard-to-contain-energy when he is not engaged in a task. It can accumulate and create a tense longing for action in him. He knows when it is there and most women easily sense its presence, though not always its innocent meanings. Feminine energy either beguiles and benefits its object for very long periods of time or has no object at all. In the latter event women also feel a storing up of inner energy and enter moments of tense need. When a woman searches for a new object she also tells the world that she will be there ever after to put her magic into it. A man tells the world that it can well believe that he will finish the job, and do more if wanted.

Yin Yang

Both kinds of energy are satisfied to support the growth of the couple's relation. This is a happy time for both. Eventually the relation is well grounded and

Your Love and His Liberty 67

the different energies begin to look outside the couple for satisfaction, and not only the male's.

The desire of the woman to securely hold the male comes up against the growing yen of the male to put energy in other places. Men tip their hand with wishes for the couple to move together around other people, events and things. Or they will wish for more directions in the relation than he to her and she to him. A sense of limitation grows, entering tension and discomfort into the relation.

Folklore sees images of jealous female possessiveness suffocating the male and of male infidelity compromising the relation. So much for folklore. The real issues involve the need for the couple to move toward more and better purpose with their energies. When the woman sees that she can trust the man, she should; and otherwise it may be time to move on. Let him know, especially without words, that he is free to follow his instincts without fear of losing you or getting less of you. Pressing him harder to be there will hold things up. Pressure stands against the easy and natural flow of his, or her, feelings to what they want and creates resentment.

Granting him liberty will result in his immediate gratitude to you. It will also leave him free to discover your meaning to him. Such honesty will leave him clear inside to sense that you are reaching to him for more of his feelings and emotions. He will want to give you more when you respect his yen to roam free at times and he will return eager to give you what you want. His motives to give will be larger than gratitude because his free time will bring him to how well suited *you* are for the good things he has to offer. He will take his liberty to mean that you understand him because you have read his inner need for action well. He will then want to do the same for you. When this is worked out by giving permission a welcome paradox sets in. The more freedom he gets, the more he discovers you and his own wish to give you more of himself. Granting liberty leads to *less* need for it and to more of emotional closeness. It also gives *you* time to clear your energy and to discover fresh things within yourself.

He will likely see you as jealous or possessive if you do not agree to his need to test his energies in new ways. Images of being limited and unreasonably controlled will overtake him and make him want time away even more. In time he will begin to detach from you. This is a situation where the communication is working but the message is not being noted. Let him be and in his free time he will find, if he cares in the first place, how he values you and wants to make your life better. This is old wisdom for many European counties. Many of the western nations follow a custom of vacationing from their relations to avoid stressing them and to keep them fresh, alive and exciting. I think they have a good idea.

I have watched these things come true for fourteen years now with a couple I know named Jane and Bob. Jane is a lively personality who seems to sense from the first that people need to feel their options, not just men. Bob puts more pride in women's abilities than most men. As they came to find each other they respected one another's special needs. I watched Bob's affections grow and deepen as he sensed Jane's support for his inner world, the world of action. Jane prospered by Bob's affectionate welcome of her abilities in all areas of life. They were each free to find more of themselves and therefore also free to love each other more. Jane sent him into life to savor his liberty with such affection that he would regularly return wanting more to be with her than by himself or with his friends, or whatever. Soon they were living together. In time they married each other. The eager love they freely gave each other continues to grow. Their love feeds off of life's challenges, making them ever closer to each other.

Your Love and His Liberty
Exercise for Chapter 8.

You will need two pieces of paper and a pen or pencil for this exercise. Draw a line down the middle of each sheet. Get comfortable and call to mind the things you want in a relation. Write them on the left side of the first sheet of paper. Now ask yourself what things you feel men want and write that on the right side. When finished put the sheet aside.

Now recall the image of a man you feel good about. He could be the one you now have a relation with or one with whom you would like to have one. Use your visualization skills to draw to you the images of his inner life of feelings, hopes and thoughts. Go into his life and world and put the second sheet before you. Now repeat the first part with <u>his</u> life experience answering for you. When you have finished compare the two sheets. How well did he answer for you and you for him? His need to be sure of your welcome affections even while away should have surfaced among his wishes.

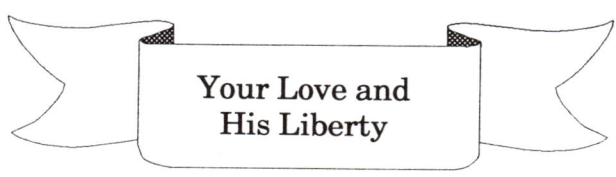

Your Love and His Liberty

Chapter 9.

Ghosts from the Past

Time present and time past
Are both perhaps present in time future,
And time future contained in time past.

...from Four Quartets. Burnt Norton
by T. S. Eliot

Remembrance and reflection how allied!
What thin partition sense from thought divide!

...from Essay on Man, epistle I by Alexander Pope

Men and women have different views on and values for their former relationships. Men hold on to them for longer periods of time than women and often return to them in their thoughts and hopes. Many wonder about the prospects of starting over again with a former love. Present hopes and fantasies of a good life are often sent to the images of former relations. Sweet and pleasant reverie follows and offers to his mind the means to a better version of the old relation.

Most find it easy for them to dispel negative memories of former relations and to muse fondly over the good things they once enjoyed. The attractive power of former relations can create a situation in which you know you are being measured against someone else. You will have an inner sense that some of him is going inward to an image whose presence is unclear to you but whose effect gives you pause. These are things that men will rarely, if ever, volunteer to you. It is a part of a man's less disclosed world that has a rightful place in your awareness.

Men carry the images of those former relations with them when looking for someone new. They form yardsticks with which to measure how good is good and how bad is bad when they come upon someone new. The same is true in each of their next relations. He will bring his former valuations to them also. There is a hope within him, especially when he is young, that you will somehow sense his wishes and make it all turn out well.

You will be alone in this. Asking him about it is likely to lead to defensive behavior and unreliable answers. Men are very unwilling to tell a woman that she in any way is not giving him enough of what he wants or needs. In their minds men have an image of a frail and vulnerable female ego that they do not want to injure.

If you think that when he looks at you there is an overlay of someone else then you are probably correct.

Ghosts from the Past

Measure the truth of the matter by how satisfying the relation is for you. Accept the offered fragments of the whole story you hope to learn as enough for your purpose.

You do not need to know it to have a healthy relation. More mature men are likely to offer some truth when asked but are more likely to assure you, lovingly, that it does not matter. They are right. It is wiser to have a better future attract you forward than to struggle against the pull of an unsatisfying past.

Women, who are more devoted from the outset, seem to send the past away much more easily. They go forward with a strong new purpose and a more eager welcome for the next person in their lives. Their way is different from men's when starting anew. You will find here another of those natural tensions between the sexes that nature put there for greater good. Its roots lie in women seeking long term and close relations while men are more tentative about relations, at least at the outset.

There is opportunity here for you to dispel the former presences that linger in his spirit. Let him see how those former presences have no hold over you and tell him without words of the good in you. If he senses that his past has a hold on you he will see you as uncommitted to your purpose and his morale will sink. The situation calls for *your natural male* energy (that's right, natural male energy). Putting yourself before him as the best he's ever had will dispel the images of the others. Do it with a high regard for yourself and he will see a natural good in you that will draw him to you.

Just after the beginning of the relation your presence will assume a parallel life in him with his visions of the past. This is something he will be quite conscious of. In his away time, when quiet and alone, he will review you and them in his mind. He will compare you and them and seek for good things in you. His purpose will be to find preference in you while keeping the images of the others. He wants to be free of his own past but he also wants to savor what it was. Let this happen without concern and it will serve your purposes and the health of the relation.

Things look differently with long term relations. If the relation lives long enough to run over and through changes in the stages of life then the images will become so faint that he will eventually part with them. This is a process that can easily take five years, and more likely ten.

He will welcome with love and gratitude the work of your presence on his inner life. The divisive hold of the past on men is ambivalent, offering both nostalgic joy and unwelcome hurt and he will therefore be glad for your help to let it go. Just don't tell him that you know. Men are more troubled by images of past relations than most women realize. That is one more reason why you are so important to the present moment of their lives.

Ghosts from the Past
Exercise for Chapter 9.

Would you like to be able to sense when images of the past are drawing him within? Find some times in your life when you were in conversation with someone but not really there. Look for those moments when a distraction invited your attention only to take complete hold of it for a while. Bring those times nearer to you so that you begin to feel lost in them. Hold the experience coming over you.

Now send your attention to the fellow you care about or one that you once did. Find some times when he made you feel as though he could have given you more of himself. Bring those times closer. Now put the experience you held in abeyance above into those images. Watch him drift away more as they work into him. How does the change in his presence affect you? Stay with the impact on you and take it with you into your life. It will be your signal that the one you are with is processing things from the past.

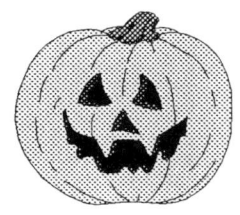

Ghosts from the Past

Chapter 10.

Ambivalence

A Woman is a foreign land,
Of which, though there he settle young,
A man will ne'er understand
The customs, the politics, and tongue.

...from The Angel in the House, by Coventry Patmore

Ambivalence reaches many parts of a man's experience of women. It is not the same variety of ambivalence as a woman's. The female's is rooted in her emotionality becoming too diffuse, making her feel without center. The male kind comes from how uninformed they become when they want to take action in the relation. Men become puzzled. A pause, different in character from the woman's, overtakes them. It can hold up a good relation or even suspend it. It may even tell you to move on and make a better choice. Most of the time, however, his ambivalence presents both of you with a variety of creative ways to improve your relation.

Men are always clear on their conscious understanding of women. They see women as the best part of life, offering heights of happiness and joy to be found nowhere else. Women are passports to higher and better states of being. At the same time men also find much about women to be past understanding and often confusing. This split reaction in men to women is intriguing in and of itself. For men it spells out an inner division of themselves that most feel they must simply learn to live with, a thing most never really succeed in doing.

Men want to be clear on their purpose. The feeling of being divided inside, with some signals going one way and others pulling oppositely, is not the comfortable and in charge kind of experience that men favor. Most males will resort to naive, brute force measures to regain a sense of directedness in their actions. Men simply have a lesser hand in the psychology of relations. Most do not feel like masters in their houses when it comes to their hearts. They usually long deep within themselves to rely on their mate to spell out what it all means.

This leads to a tension between the wish to be ready for action and the poor ability to know what to do in the first place. Men get stumped easily in relations and often just count on the flow of time to rescue them from the ambivalence of wanting to do something, anything, but not knowing what to do. They lack clear vision on themselves, the other and the relation. In other words, they have trouble seeing the whole thing.

Ambivalence tips its hand easily. Its earliest sign is usually an emphasis on its opposite: certainty. If you feel that he overstates his conviction when you talk about the relation, then you are probably correct. It is likely that you are sensing his inner struggle with his own uncertainty. Exaggerated statements of joy in the relation or on how worthwhile it is to do without other things, and so on, are telltale.

I have a friend named Ralph who is in the middle of this. He plans to marry someone he has been dating for two years. His conversation is rich in how good he feels about his upcoming marriage and how it will so benefit his life and hers. His denial of his unresolved doubts is transparent to all who care about him and who try to tell him, in a quiet way, that they should wait and learn more of one another.

After false certainty comes signs of his being off key. You will note in him some discontent with himself — not you — as he tries to deny that something is not quite right. He is still trying to hold to a former sense of satisfaction that his insides tell him is no longer there. This may be expressed as not arriving on time, less enthusiasm, distraction when with you or a general drop in the electricity of being together. You will feel the beginning of a sense of detachment that still keeps the majority of him in the relation. This is a good time to sniff out what emotional processes are trying to make their way into his conscious mind. When you find them give him an action that will help him to see what is going on.

For example, suppose you are entering a period of life where your good feeling for yourself and your self esteem is growing gingerly. At the same time he is coming to, but not yet at, a fresh challenge in his life, say nearing certification in an area that he enjoys and does well at. A good policy at this time would be to leave the amount of time you spend together up to him and to stay mindful that you will give him your good feelings in the near future.

Give him an expressed action by telling him that you want to be there with him to share what is coming up in his life. ==This will move some of the positive energy of your sense of yourself, which he sees, into the relation for sharing.== It will also energize him to go forward with you into the next piece of his life. This will give you fresh enjoyment together and preclude his feeling that he must go out and rebuild himself to keep up with you.

You will know that you have a horse of a different color on your hands when simple measures such as forced certainty and exaggeration come to their limits in helping him deal with his discontent. At the limit he will give you more open expressions of his ambivalence. This can be an "==I love you but==" scenario. It could be simpler, such as alternating between insisting on being with you, versus having to suddenly break free and be elsewhere. There is some of the latter in almost all relations at one time or another, for both sexes.

Such pronounced and easy to read ambivalence is like a fever: it tells you that the situation is either about to become much better or much worse. So stay in there and watch the omens as they unfold. If you really want this fellow and feel good about your future together then send him love and patience. On the other hand, if you feel he is not right for a relation at this time then it would probably be wiser to take time out from each other and think it through.

Ambivalence
Exercise for Chapter 10.

Part I. Here is an exercise that will bring you closer to what the male's ambivalence feels like. Take a few minutes to relax. When you feel centered give your thoughts to finding some issues you are or once were ambivalent about. Make a note of them and put them aside for the moment.

Put both your hands upon your knees with your palms down. Imagine that you are taking a perception test in which you turn your left palm up if you see yellow and your right palm up if you see red. Visualize a screen in front of you on which samples of yellow and red flash. You turns your palms as indicated.

Now imagine seeing a yellow that is closer to orange, then a red not as red but more orange than before. You move your left and right palms accordingly. The shades of yellow and red begin to so merge on the screen that you cannot distinguish the left palm signal from the right. Can you feel the difference between your right and left palms now? Do your two hands now feel like one?

Ambivalence 83

Visualize now a clear, white screen. Let your attention run freely over it. When your right and left hands again feel different move on to Part II.

Part II. Now return to the thoughts of the first paragraph in Part I. Take one part of the ambivalent issue you chose above and put it in the yellow color. Take the opposing part and put it in the red. Repeat the above seeing now one, now the other of your ambivalent parts come to you with the two colors and the palm turns they trigger. This will make you feel the male variety of (action) ambivalence come over your own.

What differences did you feel between male and female ambivalence? Does one seem more natural or desirable to you than the other?

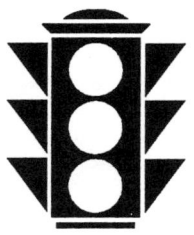

Ambivalence

Chapter 11.

Breaking Up

The beginnings and endings of all human undertakings are untidy, the building of a house, the writing of a novel, the demolition of a bridge, and, eminently, the finish of a voyage.

...from Over the River by John Galsworthy

Great is the art of beginning,
but greater the art is of ending;
Many a poem is marred by a superfluous verse.

...from Elegiac Verse
by Henry Wadsworth Longfellow

The quotes in the order given talk about the unpleasantness of an ending and the art of drawing wisdom from it. The not so nice part is shared by both the man and the woman. As for the other part, the evidence is that women leave relations with more of a will to learn from them than men. When women end a relation, romantic, social or otherwise, they are usually committed to leaving it entirely behind them and out of their lives. They may look back, especially to see, touch and understand what was, but they don't often go back. The memories, fair or foul, are usually enough for them.

Men's endings are usually less definitive. Men look back and they often go back. Men, in general, do not process the end as a definite end but more as the conclusion of an ongoing saga to which they may one day return. Nor do they tend, especially in early life, to look back to gather wisdom. One part of them looks back with warmth and sentiment to the tender moments and the closeness. This brings a sinking sense of loss to a man, a thing that men often feel has no counterpart in women. Men are often distressed by the finality with which women end relations and they often see their resolve as chilling.

The other part of men tends to coolly evaluate how successful the relation was. This is one reason, among many, why it is common for men to try to resume contact with a former relation, or even the whole thing itself. Both parts, the emotional and sentimental on the one hand, the evaluation of action on the other, live side by side in a man's spirit, perhaps reflecting a weak link in the connection of feeling to acting in men.

A woman's exit from a relation is something of the opposite of its beginning, at least with respect to how she puts in or withdraws the energy of her person. When she seeks a relation she generally intends to give a great deal of herself to it. That's the natural thing to do for a woman past adolescence or early adult life. A woman wants to send a large amount of her creative emotional energy to the relation, some doing work on her and some on him. She sets her heart and her purpose to that. She puts her hopes into creating something worthwhile with the way she plans to give herself to the relation. There is heart and feeling in this and men have little sense of the process or what it means to a woman. Men also see little of how the longing to give vital energy takes a hold of woman's insides and sends so much of her outside herself to the other. A woman in motion to build with her love is like a nation putting much capital into worthwhile commitments like roads, bridges, schools and those things that bear on the future. The woman and the nation put their own substance into their investments hoping to create enduring good.

Men also send their energy out there but not the same way. Women will select only a few objects to which they will give much love. Men will choose more objects but give them less energy. For a woman there is one great object, the man, and several lesser ones such as their home, relations and finances. This is true for both traditional and career women. A man also has that one special person but his psychological designs are different. He doesn't see her as a person to whom he is driven to send intuitive love and life creating energy. Nature's design has not put such things in his make up. He sees himself more as the architect of the relation. He wants the relation, as a thing of two, to work. His attention goes as singularly to the formation of the relation as hers goes to how their *inner worlds meet* and make it to be.

A man also has many lesser objects to which he gives his loving energy. This is true with and without a relation. It is in the nature of male energy, as noted, to go to objects that are completely formed in short periods of time. For a man only a few relations go with him through time and the rest are come and go objects offering satisfaction to his drive to make things work. The woman in his life for whom he has deep feelings is the exception.

The role of the woman he cares about in this exceptional way is unique in his life. She becomes the source of his emotional life and more and more of him goes out to meet her. When men come to care about a woman this way, they *really* care. They fall big-time, as the expression goes. The woman who becomes his emotional life outside himself has a hold over him without rival in his life.

Men suffer serious and long term hurt when a relation they are attached to this way ends. When once that lesser power to feel and sense is struck by the beautiful inner life of a woman it goes on resounding for a long time after she is gone. The lesser in him wants to remain joined to the greater in her and the loss of her is more painful to men than most women realize.

Breaking Up

The end of a relation with a woman he has come to love and to be one with emotionally is different from endings that are more casual. Here he will not think in terms of success or failure. Such reflections belong to his greater power that has been put into the background of his life. Her presence, greater where he is less, has pulled his lesser self forward to be one with her. His consciousness swims around his misty images of her emotional world and how his has become fused with it. The world of action is thrown into the remote backstage of his life while he struggles to deal with his emotional life alone, without her external life to go on creating and securing it.

This sort of reliance of him on her is a part of nature that has a parallel image in the woman. She comes to feel her inner focus and directness as his creation and his absence brings her the distress of feeling diffuse and dispersed within. Nature herself needs both forces, the male and female, and the experience of loss in relations reflects what is true of the universe itself. Like nature itself, he has the option to become more feminine in order to heal and she has the option to become more masculine in order to remain more centered.

Breaking Up
Exercise for Chapter 11.

Recall the ending of a former relation or one that you are thinking of ending. Send your imagination to the seashore. See yourself seated comfortably on a log of driftwood peering out across the water. As you listen to the rhythm of the waves you see one ship, then two. They are moving away from you, out to sea. Pick the one that is you; let the other be him. They move out away from you, first together and then apart.

Watch the one that is you pick a path in the sea that pleases you. Do likewise for him. Watch them move out and away from you and from each other. Note the weather where you sit and send them fair weather for a good and safe journey. Bid his ship farewell and continue your journey into a happy life.

Come out of the above scene and recall what in it was difficult to do. Choose such a piece of it and draw it in. Amplify everything about it, the sights, the sounds, the smells, the touches, and so on. Deepen your experience until you see what made you pause and wonder what to do.

Now turn your attention to him. Look for his sense of loss, his perceptions of the relation that disappoint you, his difficulty managing without you and so on. Go to his ship and become him looking at you on the other ship.

Hold the images for a while and let them move of their own through you. Just watch your inner experience. When you feel satisfied return to the driftwood log on the seashore and watch those ships move away from you a last time.

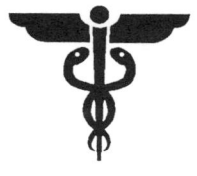

Breaking Up

Chapter 12.

Aftermath and After

Here a star, and there a star,
Some lose their way!
Here a mist, and there a mist,
Afterwards—Day!

...from No. 113 by Emily Dickinson

Once the relation is given up he will carry sweet thoughts of you with him for a long time. If he has been deeply hurt by the loss of your emotional powers he will need time to get past that inner sense of sudden loss. In time his thoughts will travel from hurt to your sweetness and to all the good things that lived in the relation. As the relation moves into the distance he will begin to look at how successful, in his eyes, the relation was. When he arrives at clarity he will place great importance on the degree of success his hindsight finds.

Unconsciously, it is otherwise. He will go assimilating you and the good of your soulful ways into himself beneath his awareness. Every now and then some completed part of this will surface into his waking thought and he will realize that it was you who created this good in him. Over a long period of time he will acknowledge all the gains in his inner world that have been the handiwork of your personality. In the short term he will have difficulty accepting how much life you gave him even though he will often muse fondly on your image.

Unless he is a man of unusual sensitivity he will have little awareness of what your aftermath is like. The sense of misinvested feeling and hope that comes over a woman after ending a relation is unfamiliar to most men. A woman returns to herself for a while and feeds off of her own feeling energy. What was once his is now put to a more immediate and personal use by her. These things are so strange to most men that the less mature ones would find a childish humor in it if they were told about it. Men, mature and otherwise, have an inner need to feel that they can always pluck up fresh bravado and go forward again into the fray. This need tends to trivialize those deeply emotional needs that are distinctive in women.

Men often show surprising outbreaks of emotion at the end of relations. Women often misread their meaning or fail to take them seriously. A man who has fallen under the spell of a woman's personality can simply feel undone when she is no longer there. He will easily lose himself in outbursts of raw emotion. Once a woman's ways open the gates of a man's emotional life they remain open and what once entered through the women now keeps flowing in her absence. But the image of her that it invited it out now lives only in his memory.

I know a woman named Elizabeth who told me about the final chapter in her recent relation. She recounted feeling at wits' end for how to respond to the emotional helplessness of her ex. He had called her shortly after their ending and was in a bad way. After two such episodes Elizabeth went from sympathy to irritation. She was dubious about his feelings. I felt that her ex was being earnest because he cared about her. She had gotten to him with her vibrant personality and awakened in him a stronger contact with himself that he ever had before. Her sudden absence left him in a lurch, almost like a novice actor who has a leading role thrust on him after performing brilliantly as an under study.

Another friend, Mary, misread the signs in an ending she went through. She took the emotionalism of her ex to signify the depth of his feeling for her. He came to her with excessive outpouring and without dignity. Mary felt that he was offering signs of a true and deep attachment to her and thought of renewing the relation. I felt that a healthy person does not compromise himself in his outreaching as her ex did and that he was trying to manipulate her back into an unhealthy relation.

In her aftermath a woman usually has other women who can help her to make sense of it all and to gather fresh energy. Women give one another support in many personal areas that men never get to. Men still do not seek out one another enough for support in personal matters. They may turn to activity, alone or with others, to move their restless sense of hurt from within to without. They use this process to unconsciously discover their meanings. While their awareness goes to something enjoyable, say hiking or travel, another part of themselves, deeper and inaccessible, is working on seeing things in a different and better way. Men accept that they will probably never have much waking contact with that part and they choose to let that part improve their lives in its own way, hidden from view.

There is a general faith in men of the power of unconscious learning and many trust it to deal with the meanings of hurt and confusion that their endings bring. In time the wisdom of a higher purpose comes over most men and they move on refreshed, going to new paths with positive images of you in their hearts. For many men the real meanings arrive in their lives as no more than pleasant inner promptings to go forward in life a certain way.

Endings have afterlives within men that can live on. They have the power to haunt when left unresolved or when too much apprehension surrounds their meaning. You will know when you are in the company of a man whose past relation still holds sway over him. It

Aftermath and After 97

begins as a sense of absence in him telling you that he has more to give if only he would choose to. The nearer you draw to him, even in the casual first conversations, the more you will feel his inner world seeking your support to reshape it for him along better lines.

Rebound is one expression of the past lingering into the present. At bottom, it is an effort to use the next person to solve the problems the last one created. A man in rebound tips his hand with a driven need to cloak his negative wish to "show her." His anger and lack of control will be close to the surface for you to read. If his past is too much present then use your ways to send him back to his issues and seek out a freer spirit to give yourself to.

Aftermath and After
Exercise for Chapter 12.

Deepen your empathy for the inner experience of loss that overtakes a man just out of a relation with a woman he had grown close to. Imagine that you are a part of an exploration into a remote region of space. It is the last of its kind. You reach your destination and come upon a higher life form who knows you. This person knows that you have always had a sense of being in the world with a special and higher purpose. You see in his eyes that he knows what it is all about.

You come to know each other and develop a relation in which love grows. Your lover's personality works on your inner life and puts you in touch with other and higher parts of yourself. Your joy and happiness grow as you draw closer to a rich part of yourself which, for all its promise, seemed so inaccessible to you. You look forward to your time together when your lover's ways reach you and give you the best moments of your life.

Your expedition is recalled and you must leave. You enter your ship with sorrow and regret. You look back from its portal to the feelings and joys written on the spacescape. You must leave the behind a wonderful part of your life. There will never be another voyage like this. You are left with the hungry memories of that other who brought you see, taste and understand some of the gifts of life waiting within you. Your life is changed for good and you can reach to the other for more only in your hopes and dreams.

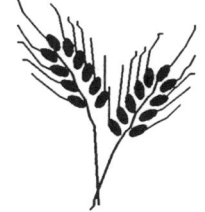

Aftermath and After

Chapter 13.

Avoidable Men

*Whatever it is, I fear Greeks
even when they bring gifts.*

...from The Aeneid by Virgil

There are men that you don't want to meet. They apply their sinister skill to plundering the advantage women have over men in the psychological area. These are men who have a highly evolved empathy for women's needs, more so than most others. Such men have a ready sense of just what a woman needs to hear or to feel. They sense what purpose a woman wants them to uphold and they offer it on the spot. They offer women instant gratification when they are most in need of it. Somewhere in the background their price is looming silently for the wary to see. They are intent on getting a rich harvest of self indulgent gains from the women they are manipulating into states of emotional blindness. *Ex: Jeff McCollum Movie: "Portrait of a Lady"*

These men have honed their craft well. Their unit of strategy is to give swift and certain emotional gain to a woman's long pent up wishes and to then swoop down on them in their moment of vulnerable gratitude. In those moments they press their claim for what they want. They press it without words in that get-my-message emotional way that women cannot miss. Their wants are not among the most admirable choices men can have.

Sexual favor is the most obvious want a man can have. It is not the easiest good to manipulate his way into despite the general conviction going the other way. A man who seeks a woman who like himself wants a sexual tryst does not have to look very far. He is not the man depicted here. This man goes after the sexual favors of women who set considerable value by their affections and intimacies.

The challenge is to wrest that tenderness from one who is not so willing to give it. He is vigilant for the virtuous maiden in distress, so to speak, and she is his easy prey. After his satisfactions he tips his hand with sudden loss of interest and a pull to other, more pressing things in his life. When he returns he will once again be concerned with his needs and highly attentive to hers. And she may fall for it a second time, and a third time, and so on.

Watch out for him. Insincerity is his trademark and he wears his it on his nose. How will you know him when you see him? He will be overly attentive to things that are so, so important to you and so eager to bring you to drink an easy and deep draft of what you want. A woman who values the gift of herself and who is just out of a relation is vulnerable to this. So is a guilty woman with a need to be hurt, another trait he will easily pick up on.

You can test this fellow by inviting him to something that calls for authenticity and sincerity. For example, suggest how nice it would be to meet your married sister and their budding family. Or an invitation to meet your support group is sure to make him tense. You can also call him out by testing for where he places his values and suggest that he meet your sister the therapist or your brother the attorney. You can call his bluff from the other end by feigning interest in insincere relations, a thing you can casually reveal in your emotional messages and conversation. If he comes at you like a peer in these matters you will know that you have found him out.

There is a worse nuisance to women than the immature man taken with Don Juanism. He is driven by what may first pass as a charming immaturity within him. He wants you to arrange his world for him, and everything else. His bright and creative energy goes not to taking care of himself but to taking care of selected needs in you that make you so, so willing to take care of him. Clinicians would say that he is the man with unresolved dependency. His instincts are soft and gentle and his ways are benign. Often he will be almost saintly. Always he will make you feel guilty for even thinking of not giving him what he needs. The image of a child will come to you when you see him but you will want to put it away when you see the power of his imaginative and sensual ways. How could you know that those talents do not go out to solve the ordinary problems of life? You can know if you sensitize yourself to look for his personality style.

The boyish ways of such a man can seem to be a guarantee of secure safety with him. That is surely true in most of the areas you would want to safeguard. The hazard here is that he may turn into a black hole for your energy and devotion and may leave you psychologically hungry in many ways. What becomes of your healthy yen for a man to make you feel centered and well oriented within yourself? To whom do you turn when you want more of the emotional energy and ways of the other sex? Most of the ordinary short-term snares in a relation are guaranteed to <u>not</u> happen with this sort of man but many others, of a longer term character, are <u>guaranteed</u> to happen.

Barring the obvious there is yet a more avoidable kind of man that you don't want in your life. Psychiatry refers to his problem as narcissism. This is a fellow who is very much taken with himself. He can be quite intriguing and often colorful in the way he invites you to enter the wonder of his world. His personality style is highly seductive and often not in a sexual way, though that usually comes later. He wants you in his orbit adoring him and finding joy in what he regards as his great beauty and magnificence.

Paradoxically this fellow can usually also give a great deal of love. Problems arise more from the way he frustrates the good of the relation rather than you. The more you adulate him the more he will give you love and tenderness but not the kind that serves coming together and getting closer. His love is more like a congratulation with sex added. This is a devilish personality because this fellow will usually be bright, informed and accomplished. It is easy to fall under his spell and to lose a great deal of time wishing for better from him. It won't come. His love is centered on himself and only a limited amount of it really goes out to others.

He is not a fellow who poses obvious risks like the others. The risk here is that he will pull so much love and hope out of you that when you finally realize that it will never go anywhere you will feel drained and exhausted. The aftermath can hold you up a long time while you mend and get perspective. It's a sticky wicket because while you are with him you will probably feel wonderful — just like he feels about himself.

This fellow is easy to spot despite the subtlety of the risks involved in being with him. He will have a sophisticated flair in his style and you will feel oh so drawn to him. He is sure to look upscale and like a part of the good life. And then the telltale sign, his grandiosity, will ooze from his pores. Look carefully when you meet him because he can enchant you with his go nowhere ways and make you want to stay with him a long, long time.

Avoidable Men
Exercise for Chapter 13.

This will help you to see if you are drawing the kind of men you would rather avoid. Get a piece of paper and a pen or pencil. Draw a line down the middle. Create a mental image of each of the avoidable men described: the high rolling Don Juan, the clinging take-care-of-me lover, and the self inflated narcissist. Let the images move freely and draw your feelings out. Note the words that come to mind and write them on the left side of the paper. Record also any words that repeat as you move from image to image.

When you have finished do a clearing exercise. Imagine everything you just did going backwards to before you began this exercise. Now imagine a place you want to be at with someone special. Go to it and savor the experience. Muse over the person you are with and feel your emotions going out to meet him. Record on the right side of the paper the words that come to mind in this experience.

Count the number of words you used to describe the avoidable men and the number used to describe what you wish for. Which is greater and what does the greater number tell you about your goals? For each of the three kinds of avoidable men count the number of words that describe him and that also occur on the right side of the paper. How large a fraction of what you look for is it? Add up the last three numbers and compare it to the right hand total. What does this figure tell you about how much your unconscious images are looking for someone who may not be so good for you?

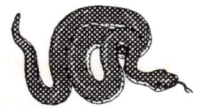

Avoidable Men

Chapter 14.

Things Men Dream About

"The game's going on rather better now," she said, by way of keeping up the conversation a little. "'Tis so," said the Duchess: "and the moral of that is —'Oh, 'tis love, 'tis love, that makes the world go round!'"

...from Alice's Adventures in Wonderland
by Lewis Carroll

A mans's dreams are much more on the moments where he and his wish come together than on what happens afterward. He assumes in his hopes that if he and she can meet as he wants then all else will follow. It may bring dismay to hear that a man's dreamy focus is much more on the time of meeting than on the sexual passion that may follow, but it is so. It is so because so much of his time and energy is used to rehearse making that one special but crucial moment work, the moment where the one before him will favor him as much as he does her.

His heart, soul and mind are full of hopes that he will meet someone who will draw his person to hers. He hears the voice and sees the gestures of the ideal woman he has in mind and he puts their images into the very first time you both meet. His reverie lingers on those moments of sweet first encounter where he discovers certain wished for things in you and little goes to the good things he will later enjoy with you.

In their hearts men wish for a woman who will be what they regard as reasonable, a trait they feel certain will manifest itself from the very first. This wish is for a variety of shared action that presupposes your reading his signals well, those things he says and does that communicate his meaning and intentions along the lines of doing more than feeling. He makes his ideal image vivid with themes of emotional cooperation.

Men steel themselves before they approach women because they know how highly women prize their gifts. They anticipate that a woman will first want to see much of value in him and perhaps hide her positive feelings for his advance. What's on the man's mind is that this is the moment and if you don't take it then it will probably be lost for good. Men *feel* that women, even women who are interested in their advances, place more value on inner ideals of propriety and courting ritual than on the practical issue of meeting. This leads, in a man's view, to satisfying those values at the risk of losing the opportunity to connect with him. This issue is a deep concern for most men. They are apprehensive that their best efforts can easily fail to connect even when the woman they desire so much is interested in him.

> In the man's mind, the *ideal* woman will help a man when he tries his luck with her. She would make it clear, in terms he understands, that she is interested in his flirtation. How do you do that? Begin with an obvious smile and then offer an easy to read reply such as "You're interesting. I'd like to hear more about you." This translates in a man's mind as "she is telling me that she likes what I do to her and that she wants to spend some time together." Men dream probably every day of women who will do such things as this. Believe it. The woman who is willing to work to spare a man the efforts he has grown accustomed to undertake, and with not enough return in his eyes, will go very, very far with men.

I had an experience some time ago along these lines that is memorable. I was in a shopping mall seated under some lovely trees and writing out a greeting card. Seated across from me was an attractive woman whom I noted and had an inner wish to learn more about, given the obvious charm of her appearance and manner. She looked my way and made her interest clear. When I realized that I had no stamp for my card I knew what to do — I asked her if she had one. She searched about and found one that I purchased from her. We began to talk about my greeting card which, as it happens, was especially humorous and therefore served my purpose to show her. When I began to walk back to my seat to post my greeting card, she came with me.

We resumed our conversation there and she gingerly went back to where she had been seated to get the rest of her belongings. She made it so easy to see, without compromising her dignity, that she wanted to talk and see what I was I like. She also made it clear that she welcomed my obvious interest in her. She did it right and very much the way men hope women will.

The particulars of men's dreams are similar and are far more psychological as opposed to sexual than women tend to assume. Making it easier to meet is an example of a larger wish in men for women who will make their meanings obvious through action and not only through feelings. Men call this being reasonable though most would be hard put to express their wish in words. Men do not decode feelings as readily as actions. Send them messages in action or in things that suggest action and they will get your meanings and see you as the one to be with.

How do you suggest action? Talk about the things you do with relish and enthusiasm. It doesn't matter what they are because a man will pick up on the element of doing and of feeling good about doing. He will take those items to contain the messages and will tend to miss most of the other emotions you send him in what you say. For example, tell him about the rush of feeling and energy you get when you down hill ski, or about the excitement of horseback riding, or of how dynamic a speaker was (rather than the topic) and so on. He will listen for the doing and the energizing involvement rather than the inner emotional response. He will look for things in your narrative that pull his energy out to the particulars of action and the excitement of doing, as opposed to living, the event.

As for the sexual ideal itself, there is little in the way of surprise. Men who are thin want thin women with attractive faces and heavier men want heavier women. Different personal stories and chemistries make for a great deal of variety in preference for one part of the figure over another. Every man would like a beautiful woman but that's not the end of the story. Dwelling on surface appearance can limit and even block sensitivity to the other things men wish for that are usually more important to them. Men are much more in tune with the feelings you give them than anything else you offer. Men do not understand feelings as easily or as deeply as women but they respond to what your feelings do to them whether or not they know their meanings.

There is only one physical trait that men set great store on with any uniformity. That one trait is *comfort*. It means what it says. A man wants to feel physically comfortable when he is close to you, as when he dances with you, holds you and certainly when he makes love to you. You can create some of this comfort by getting a sense of his body movements. The more you flow together and well align yourselves the more comfortable he will find you — and want to be near you. It is remarkable how many men decide a woman's comfort by the way she feels in a slow dance. He will find you comfortable when your places near one another are easily found and so make you flow as one.

Most of what remains in his ideal is more abstract than emotional. Men want to think that the ideal opening scene heralds more of the same in the relation. They want being with you and getting to know you to be open and shared and active. They want your life to come easily into them and they want to feel important to you. The wish so pervasive in women, to make a man happy, is also in men. They want to feel that they bring light and joy to the woman they care about. Their ability to do this for *her* is an important part of *his* interaction with that ideal, wished for woman.

When a man feels that he makes a woman glow with joy for his sake it puts to rest a nagging anxiety in him. Men who see that the woman they love also is taken with them have that same worry in the back of their minds as women. It is the fear that her joyous regard for him will one day no longer be there. Men and women meet on a common ground of concern in this matter. You would be ideal with that fellow you love, or want to love, if your spirit goes to him freely and openly, with an easy and natural elan that tells him what it's all about. Men love that and you will love what they give you in reply to it.

Things Men Dream About 115

The giving, as opposed to the getting, part of sex also belong to the ideal. Men's longing for their own sexual gain has grown into a fiction of mythic size. Their sexual drive can be impulsive but their interest in women, especially when they have a relation in mind, goes beyond just passion. Most men will respond to a woman's feeling that his interests are limited to sex with disappointment and sometimes resentment. They know that their intentions and goals go to more things than just making love. When a man cares for a woman it becomes important to him to show it by bringing joy and happiness to her life. When he cares enough to want to care more then he will want to give the relation the tenderness it needs to grow and deepen. A woman's satisfaction is important to him and by more than most women may at first assume.

To him making love is the highest form of shared action you can have together. He may not consciously realize it in words but that is how he functions. In those tender moments he makes his meanings known to you in a preferred and natural way. He will read what he means to you by how much your affections make him feel that you are connected to him. Men assume that if you care about them, you will then want to give each other those ecstatic and remarkable joys found only in lovers' trysts. A man's ideal lover is a woman who welcomes his affections and who openly shows her love in the way she makes love. Lovemaking assures a man both of your affection and of your willingness to be on his side, so to speak, in all of life. Most men assume that they can measure the degree to which a woman will be this way by how she receives him when they first meet. The idea of easy and natural communication expressed in eagerly shared activity is in the man's mind from the very first.

Things Men Dream About
Exercise for Chapter 14.

This is a Pygmalion and Galatea exercise. Imagine a man like Pygmalion devoting his creative energy to sculpting the ideal woman. Let yourself be his ivory figure of that perfect woman Galatea. Draw Pygmalion to you and feel his passion go out to sculpture the form and suggestive lines of that ideal woman. Feel the soul he is putting into her with every gentle stroke of his mallet. Step into Pygmalion. Feel his hands sending his ideal form into the figure of Galatea. Your eyes are his eyes. You study the statue of Galatea and you see your hands remove what hides that ideal woman there beneath the ivory. What do his eyes see and what are his hands trying to depict? Breathe the hope and longing of Pygmalion.

Now go to Galatea. Become one with the object of his love and dreams. Look to your sculptor and see his fiery passion to bestow perfect and ideal life on you. Each mallet blow comes to you with vibrant and life giving energy, shearing away the smallest imperfection. You feel the heat of his hands and face near you and you see the form he wishes for in you. You are Galatea the ideal woman of Pygmalion. What does the form he gives you mean to him?

Now go to real life. Recall a relation, not one you are presently in. Give the role of Pygmalion to him and of Galatea to yourself. Now work the images of this exercise into yourself and him and compare what you sense and feel with what you experienced when you were in the relation. You can use this exercise to go forward sensitized to the ideal that men search for and bring it to your present or next relation.

The myth of Pygmalion and Galatea comes to a charming close. Pygmalion longs for the perfection of his ivory statue to come to life. Venus is touched by his wish and grants it. Pygmalion names his ideal come to life Galatea. Pygmalion and Galatea love each other and grow a life together.

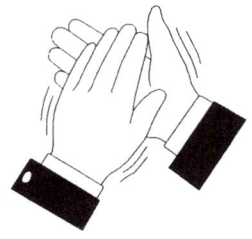

Things Men Dream About

Chapter 15.

The Women Men Fear

In what distant deeps or skies
Burnt the fire of thine eyes?
On what wings dare he aspire?
What the hand dare seize the fire?

...from The Tiger by William Blake

Most of women's powers over men are rooted in what poets have called the eternal feminine, a wonder of nature promising men a joy and happiness unlike anything else life has to offer. Men easily lose themselves to the awesome power women have to put such a great goodness into them. They easily generalize to everything else a woman offers and, especially when they are young, they fail to note the things they later learn to guard against. They soon learn to make a study of separating the chaff from the wheat. Getting past the emotions that overtake them in women's presence and arriving at clear judgment soon becomes an issue in their lives.

The lure of a beautiful woman can easily take hold of a man and put his good senses behind him, at least for a while. Why then is it that the more beautiful a woman is the fewer the men who approach her? Women, other than the one in question, usually assume that men so fear rejection that they would rather take no chances. It looks differently through a man's eyes. The first thing a man has anxieties for is that she will bargain too hard emotionally because of her beauty. That is, men expect that pretty lady to be pretty hard to please. That expectation is so great that most men avoid her. They feel more inclined to more easily, in their eyes, win the enjoyable affections of one not so beautiful but more accessible.

The pretty lady whom no one approaches rouses an anxiety that puts men off. They may well be in error for avoiding her but the signal anxiety driving them away is real. Other women, more inclined to direct and define the relation, pique that anxiety even more. It is an anxiety announcing that he will have to work long and hard to get close enough for even small portions of the affections and other emotional goods that relationships are meant to offer. It tells of a dark bargain where the woman will win her satisfactions at too much of a cost to the man.

There are unhealthy men who want to take part in this sort of relation. They are said to be sadomasochistic, meaning that they enjoy being made to suffer. They are not among mental health's fair haired children. Most men know enough to avoid it, and carefully too. There are a host of unsavory emotional cues that are exchanged between such a woman and the man before her. Feeling messages go out from her telling him that he must be willing to submit if he is to have a involvement with her. He senses the angry, frustrating forces that move her spirit and make her delight in depriving him of a full measure of satisfaction. She senses, unconsciously, that he will feed off of the privations. Two people meet and collude unconsciously to take part in a dance of mutual unhealth, one doling out an exciting form of emotional pain and the other welcoming it.

Nature has put a wisdom in men that knows the truer meaning of it all. A robust and deeply intuitive voice in men tells them the higher purpose of women is wonderfully creative. He knows that her first instincts are to give and uphold life. Men's inner eye sees that the woman who stirs a certain anxiety is acting against her own purpose. The deepest reason for healthy men to pause before such a woman is the innate, usually unconscious, sense that she is working against the meaning of her nature. At bottom a man perceives an opposing tension in the woman between her intuitive, creative makeup and her choice to go against it in some ways.

Most men are well enough along to sense that a woman's energies are not all moving with her higher purpose. They know, part by inner wisdom and part by rueful experience, how to read the omens. Gestures of eye, mouth and facial expression often reveal a devilish delight in mixing pain and pleasure. This can make for a healthy and enticing mixture that comes across as sexy, and actually is. Unhealth is where the ingredients are not properly mixed or in the wrong proportions. It tells in certain of the woman's ways. She will show a waiting hunger for pleasure in giving and receiving the right kind of pain. Her attention will easily go to people with ambivalence and inner tension. She watches with excitement people caught in clashes of power, hoping to find better ways to dominate and win control by studying the ways of the winner. She is thrilled by the prospect of looming danger and what frightens others will entice her.

Her pride is vested in the idea of acquiring more emotional slaves. Her inner sense of misaligned power betrays itself in the mastery she has not over herself but over those who submit to her. Measure her self esteem by how well she disowns the need for affectionate ties to men and by how completely she tyrannizes their emotional needs. Men know her well and know well how to avoid her. Her presence brings an eerie shudder to most men and they move on sensing that more and better is to be found elsewhere.

Men want from women the blessings of that other voice of nature they have less of. And, in like manner, they want the voice they have more of to work for good in women. They want more than meager portions of that unique warmth and welcome mystery so abundant in women. They sense the stifling of their spirit sure to follow in the company of women who begrudge rather than bestow their emotional richness. And they will move quickly past the woman who makes them struggle for her affections to another who will offer a more temperate spirit.

The Women Men Fear
Exercise for Chapter 15.

This exercise will help you to work better with the meaning of men's apprehensions. Bring to mind some men you have known who made you feel concerned about your interaction with them. A man whom you sensed had trouble dealing with his feminine side might be one. If you cannot recall any then try some of images from the movies or television. Use visualization to reconstruct your encounter with him and to bring it close in to you.

You will probably feel images of flight coming over you. Go with the image that pulls you away and follow its lead wherever it takes you. Stay with it until motion stops. Where are you? Have you landed in some idyllic place with a bountiful nature around you? If so you probably began with an image of frustration. Have you come to a pleasant place with a beautiful and welcome climate? If so then it is likely that you began with images of anger. Use the content of the final scene to work backwards to the feeling that brought you there.

Now choose one of the ideas from this chapter and follow the images it brings to you. Use visualization to step into a man's experience of concern. Repeat the procedure in the paragraphs above and get to the meaning of his feelings. When you are finished clear your energy by allowing yourself to follow any favorable image that comes to mind. Go with it to its end and stay there until you feel a restless urge to move on.

The Women Men Fear

Chapter 16.

Sex

To men a man is but a mind. Who cares
What face he carries or what form he wears?
But woman's body is the woman. O
Stay thou, my sweetheart, and do never go.

...from The Devil's Dictionary by Ambrose Bierce

The signs are everywhere that women have a larger share of the common purpose to create life. A man's spirit see her life giving energy and goes out to welcome it. Men know well that a woman's surface beauty is a small hint of the greater marvel within her. Women set off major movements in men telling of riches that move past the natural limits of language. Nature has given everyone feelings and emotions that know these things at once even if they are unable to put them into words. The sense of awe, the ethereal, the immortal and the limitless are true to what nature is. These things are the common joy of all lovers, and lovers know their meaning at many levels.

Lovers easily become lost in the dreaminess of their lovemaking. The experience is like an altered state in which they forget where they are and lose sense of time. It draws them on creating both more of pleasure and of a unique tension that promises still more pleasure. A man looks at his lover and his eyes move past her entrancing beauty to another and more spellbinding beauty in her person. He knows the meaning of what she does to him only in the way it transports him. He sees the universe in her and passes through her into other dimensions. The things in her person knowable to him only by her closeness alter him more each time they make love.

He leaves her reluctantly at some later time and the sweet and cloudy images of the precious time together continue to work on his spirit. His energy is drawn to what he finds in her. He cannot usually put it in words but he knows enough to enjoy the quick flow of himself to her image within him. He knows also that her image brings him a larger feeling for the generative forces of the universe than he could have alone.

The act and art of sex creates more of himself through her. Each time a man makes love he becomes more like the one he loves. Women seem to have a better grasp of this as in most matters psychological. They seem to be comfortable with being a source of life to him and somehow they tap into a vital and life giving energy for *themselves* by doing so. It can only be an energy that puts them closer to what is at the heart of nature, a thing women have a more ready sense of. Men are not often aware of the wonders a woman receives in love making, beyond the obvious, but they know very well how her affections go to work on themselves. Men can simply become undone by how attached they become to women, and more so than vice versa.

For many centuries the greater power of sex had the lesser voice in human affairs. It was portrayed as the way to children and family. Its irresistible sway over lovers was trivialized as adolescent and sure to dissolve quickly away leaving behind forlorn and dismayed lovers. The world is now standing up to a truer vision of it all. The greater power is the power to make one of two. In it each comes nearer to the way of other and both become more. The romantic tradition rightly points to the lovers' happiness in fulfilling one another.

Lovemaking as the highest form of shared action is closer to his consciousness than the ways in which her psyche enters and transforms him. He will see that shared action in all your other times together. He is far more capable of measuring meaning by its presence in action than in feeling. And so the afterlife of lovemaking will go unnoted in him except by the growth in his sense of well being and happiness. Many of the meanings in it will likely pass him by but he will know

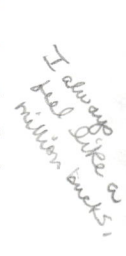

I always feel like a million bucks!

how good it makes him feel and that will draw him on for more and more of the wonders he finds in you. Some few come to realize that a woman works them into the more effective bearers of action they wish to be.

He will want to see that you are satisfied in your intimate time together. Getting to the moments of your intense and shared pleasure are important to him; issues of technique wait and serve that higher priority in his mind. Those moments tell him that you work well together and he will then feel connected to you. If you try to tell him of the meanings in what you feel together, he will probably give you an admiring smile and see you as more lovable for your ways. He is not likely to get it but he will happily accept that you are closer in what you are to many of the deeper meanings of the intimacy you have together.

He wants you to know that your sexual time together means more to him than only pleasure. Men who care are sensitive to women reducing their joy in sex to no more than mechanics. If you know that there is meaning in his lovemaking you will need to do more than to feel it because of how he reads messages. Support his weaker ability to see your messages in your feelings with an expression he will understand. Show him your meaning with mirth and merriment. Tease him with something like "Well, do you want to fool around again" or better "Do you have a headache again tonight?" He will get the message. In a man's mind humor is a form of expressed action. He will respect you and value you more for putting your sensual wishes into wit and caprice because that satisfies several of his wishes at the same time.

Sex
Exercise for Chapter 16.

Part I. Find out more about how aware you are of shared action in your love life. Find some material in your life that expresses emotion in a clear and easy to see way. Pick one and go close to the images to find a color that you associate with it. Note the color. Now use material from your life that makes action equally easy to see. Repeat the procedure to find a color that you link to the expressed action. If the two colors agree then examine their texture for difference or some other quality which sets them apart.

Picture a white screen on which images can appear only in grey (if your feeling or action colors are black or white use a different screen color). Get some images of lovemaking with your present or a former lover. Put those images on the screen so that they appear in grey. Now pigment what you see with your feeling color and let the scene unfold. What do you find coming over you now as the feeling part of lovemaking? Does it differ from what you expected? Repeat this with the color for action.

Carry this exercise a step further. Use a photo or other picture of the man you had in mind. Study it, touch it and hold it until it makes your time with him feel real and present. Repeat the coloring exercise above. What was different this time when you began with his photo?

Part II. Now redo Part I as him. First spend a few moments visualizing his inner experience. When it seems rich enough to overtake you step into it. Redo Part I in *his* shoes. Was there a shift in the choice of feeling and action colors? What does he value in his feelings and in what he does? Is there more or less feeling material in his role? What can you say about the amount of expressed action — more or less?

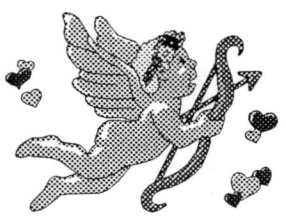

Sex

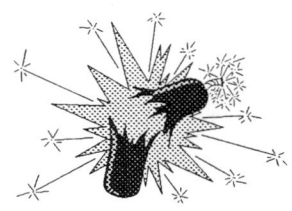

Chapter 17.

Lady Godiva

Forward and frolic glee was there,
The will to do, the soul to dare.

...from The Lady of the Lake
by Sir Walter Scott

Lady Godiva is a romantic figure whose image in this century continues to gather more and more favor among men. She elicits feelings of admiration that are well past the seductiveness in the image of a nude, beautiful woman straddling a powerful horse. The real Lady Godiva was an English countess in the eleventh century. She is portrayed as a woman with considerable sympathy for ordinary people, a trait around which legends grew, bringing her posthumous fame.

Legend and folklore have it that she appealed to her husband Leofric, the Earl of Leicester, to lift the burden of oppressive taxes from the people of Coventry. She kept after Leofric unrelentingly and became something of a nuisance to him. He then tried to put her off with an offer to ease the taxes provided that she ride nude on horseback through the town of Coventry. She accepted the challenge and astonished everyone concerned. She hid her considerable physical beauty by letting her hair down so that only her legs and face were visible when riding on the horse. Later legend has it that the townspeople, and especially the men, were sheltered from view behind shuttered windows. The figure of Peeping Tom also crept in later, perhaps securing the lesser, seductive part of her story.

The legend is charming and draws a hearty and favorable response from most men. Their response to her daring tells much about their hopes for women. Lady Godiva's legendary act puts attention on her courage to act for a higher cause and makes little note of her sexuality beyond her beauty. At a time of rigid male dominance she confronted authority for being unreasonable and out of sympathy with ordinary people. In the legend that formed around her personality, she chose to defy the rigid attitudes on sex and morality of her day in order to bring economic relief to many.

Put differently, here is a woman who put her traditional sexual role aside, flaunted moral prudence and male authority and who chose to fight for a cause rich in social purpose. Today she would be called a feminist and today she is held in high regard by most men. They see in her a richer and better hope for women, a hope rooted in the prospect of her taking action.

Most men want women who can do. It is a part of the shared action that means so much to men in relations.

Here is a cultural affirmation of what most men want for women. Men may not be able, in general, to find the words for why their feelings of support and adulation go out to Lady Godiva, but those heartfelt emotions tell a truth about their makeup. Men cannot help wanting to see their drive for directed action come to life in women. Their sympathy adds a spirit of fair play to everything else that women bring out in them. The way men feel about her story speaks well of and with great hope for what men want in their relations with women. Lady Godiva is both the beauty of the eternal feminine and the focused purpose of male action, with chutzpa thrown in.

She has become a recurring figure in life symbolizing feminine strengths that men once took too little note of. In her saga it is her husband Leofric who suggests that she do something that could only be unthinkable at that time. His parry to her is interesting because she chose to act for the common good, a moral issue, and he replies with an insult to the common good by offering an immoral option. In other words, Leofric knowing her character thought he had her painted into a corner from which she could not budge. Lady Godiva undoes his strategy of appeal to convention with a valor that outclassed Leofric by taking his dare. She had him, not vice versa! She wins by sending ethical strength to support her sensitivity and higher purpose. Leofric's insult to her first appeal energizes Godiva to appeal to an even higher and greater good than she began with. Her strength of purpose gave Leofric no other option than to concede.

The precedent of her legend is now almost a millennium old. She adds balance to the idea of what a woman is and can be. Her image suggests a rich feminine beauty joining the other side of her own nature by taking action to realize a higher purpose. Her daring do seasons her loveliness giving men an image that draws them to her. They see in her the things they want of a woman and some of the things they want in themselves.

Lady Godiva
Exercise for Chapter 17.

Here is an exercise to help you feel how much men give their hearts in support of women's wishes. Think of a male reporter for whom you have positive feelings. He should ideally be a reporter who admires women who can. If there are none make one up, like Clark Kent perhaps. Step into his experience.

You travel across time to the eleventh century to report on the day of Lady Godiva's ride through Coventry. Everyone in the town but you is behind closed doors. She approaches gently on horseback and sees you watching her and noting all that she does. She is puzzled but not dismayed. You explain why you are there and your eyes and gestures give her your admiration. She believes you and accepts your reason for being there. She invites you to traverse the town together because you trust in her purpose. She tells you the entire story behind her ride — your scoop! You are drawn together by faith in each other's purpose. You note all these things and she then sends you back to your own time to tell of them.

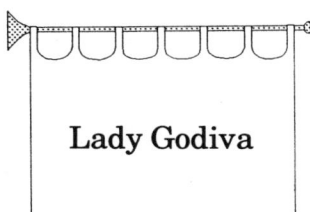

Lady Godiva

Chapter 18.

Knowing How Men See You

*Mirrors should reflect a little
before throwing back images.*

...from Des Beaux-Arts by Jean Cocteau

Nature has generously provided for each sex to have all it needs to understand the other — with a little spicy work, that is. Part of her mysterious design is to lure everyone into relationships as a means of discovering and bringing to life the rest of themselves. You should go forward with confidence that every wish to understand the other reflects your becoming able to have what you want. There is within you a full image of the male and within him is a full image of the female. You are a woman because the feminine principle is the stronger in you and he is a man because the masculine principle is the stronger in him. You both have inner outlines of each other's basic makeup.

Nature wants the other gender in you to come to life. Its growth brings joy, power and well being. It grows best in the close company of the other sex. When your love life is not going so well cheer up because it means that you and he have an opportunity. Go to the issue in your mind's eye and draw to yourself images of his ways. This will awaken in you the masculine part of yourself to match his and will bring you the inner understanding that you as a woman find natural. Use visualization to step into his personality and then try to see yourself as he does. Stay here until you feel an urge to go to the next paragraph.

You are now primed to go deeper into his experience. Keep the issue in mind and look at the last page of this chapter (p. 146). The upper two circles on the top of that page are filled in with words for the style of how men see life and the world. The imagery suggests two eyes. Put the palm of your left hand over the left hand circle of words and likewise for the right palm. Let your palms rest there while you let the issue move freely through you.

When you feel centered lift your palms up and put your fingers in the circles. Look at the words as you do this. Let them move freely to whatever words draw them. When your fingers have settled somewhere look at the words they point to. Use those key words to look at the issue through his eyes and with his masculine personalty style. Let some images form around what you feel. Note what they are and move on.

The lower circle on the final page has words for the meaning, or content, of the issue. It may help you to think of it as representing a mouth whose voice will give you his meaning. A dashed line splits the circle in two, the left side being roughly issues that are negatively charged in him and the right positively charged. Put your right hand over the circle (if left handed use your left hand). Let your hand move slowly and gently over the words in it. The sense of the words will speak to your touch. When you feel your fingers or palm come to rest look at the key words they are on. Use them to describe what the issue means to him. Allow some images to grow around what you see and feel.

Now use both sets of words that you selected. Simultaneously use your left hand to touch the key words in the upper circle(s) and your right hand to touch the key words in the lower circle. Let the images of those words from the above paragraphs come to you.

Visualize them entering you through each arm and meeting and mixing within you. His perception of the issue flows from your left and meets with what it means to him from your right. You feel his style and his sense of what you wish to resolve. Take your understanding with you as reenter the places and scenes where the issue arose. Go to the issue with a deeper understanding of his experience and energy to rework it for the better.

Knowing How Men See You
Exercise for Chapter 18.

Prepare yourself for your future. Pick something you like very, very much. It could be a favorite food, a color, a piece of music or whatever. Note what it is and put it aside for the moment. Now imagine something between you and the fellow you care about or are interested in that you want to see more clearly. It is important for this to be a fiction, so make this up.

Put the make believe issue on a screen in front of you. Imagine that your eyes are looking at the screen through the two upper word circles on page 146 (his eyes). Now add to that the image of your voice speaking through the lower word circle (his voice). Hold this image.

Now recall that something that you like very, very much. Put its image on the screen and use the eye and voice imagery above to look at it and talk about it. When in your future something surfaces that you want to see through his eyes recall your favorite something on the screen and the images of sight and speech that it carried. Then put the issue's image on the screen in its place. You now have an inner way to discover how he sees you.

After you have done this exercise a few times you will see how much you get to know about him. Do it often, as the need arises to get clear on how he sees the same thing.

You and your relationship will prosper as your sense of how he sees you grows. You will awaken more life within you by taking on his eyes and his energy. Season your first image of yourself with his. Knowing how he sees you will show you how to get more of what you want in your life. Here are my good wishes for you and for the better love you will create in your life.

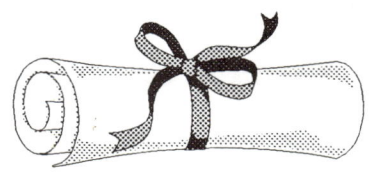

Knowing How Men See You

Knowing How Men See You

active directed
risky planned centered bold
effective hardy reasoned male
ambivalent steady clever sexy
husky scientific pragmatic
aggressive puzzled

dynamic focused
objective logical free smart
hearty expressed impulsive cute
practical vigorous daring loving
energetic dedicated reserved
ambitious intrepid

Through His Eyes

control	:	admire
stagnate exploit	:	fulfill grow
avoid hurt disregard	:	nurture awaken close
flee plunder persecute	:	support hearten energize
manipulate hurt limit	:	uplift enjoy reveal engage
wound ignore remote	:	empathize trust uphold
depress thwart	:	discover realize
suspect	:	sympathize

Darker Intention : *Lighter Intention*

Dear Reader:

Thank you for reading HOW TO HAVE YOUR WAY WITH MEN. Your comments on it are welcome. Send them to:

>Scientific Support
>19 Crest Street
>Westwood, NJ 07675.

Order additional copies of HOW TO HAVE YOUR WAY WITH MEN by sending $15.00, check or money order, to Scientific Support at the above address or call 201-358-8754 anytime.

Best wishes to you!